THROUGH THE WORDS OF 400 INTERNATIONAL
RESEARCH PARTICIPANTS

Have They Gone
Nuts?

**The Survival Guide to Social Interaction
in Neurodiverse (Autistic-Neurotypical)
Relationships**

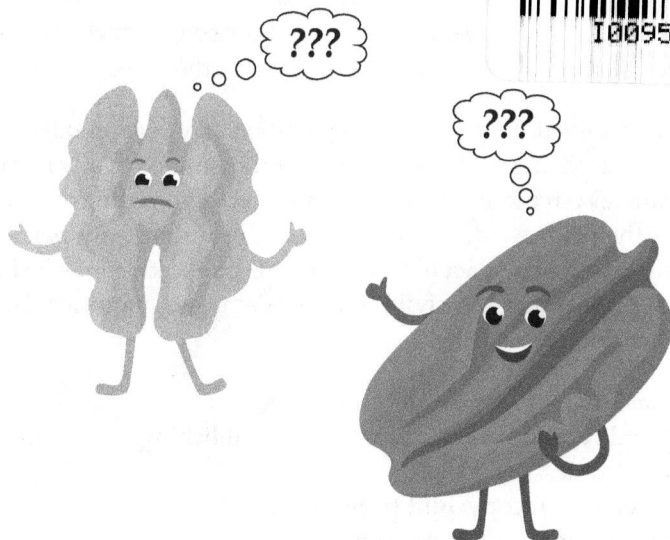

Dr Bronwyn Maree Wilson
Foreword by Professor Tony Attwood

First published by Ultimate World Publishing 2022
Copyright © 2022 Dr Bronwyn Wilson

ISBN

Paperback: 978-1-922828-20-0
Ebook: 978-1-922828-21-7

Cover design: Ultimate World Publishing
Layout and typesetting: Ultimate World Publishing
Editor: Marinda Wilkinson
Cover illustration copyright license:
Andrii Bezvershenko-Shutterstock.com

Ultimate World Publishing
Diamond Creek,
Victoria Australia 3089
www.writeabook.com.au

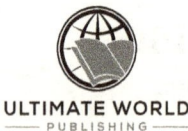

Testimonials

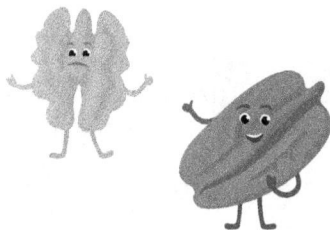

I am very much looking forward to reading all three of your soon-to-be published books. As I've mentioned before, your dissertation had an immense impact on my thinking about the influence of my father's Asperger's on the dynamics of my family's behaviours. Your study has totally shifted my attitude of hatred to one of understanding and compassion for the man who helped bring me into this world.

I'm serious when I say that reading your dissertation turned my world upside down. I had held such anger in my body and mind about my father's behaviours that I was frankly relieved when he finally died four hours short of his one hundredth and one birthday. I had known zilch about Asperger's until I read your dissertation and began to figure things out about the dynamics in my family of origin.

Dr Ann List,
American school Social Worker

Have They Gone Nuts?

Have They Gone Nuts? 'IS' the book that will help relationships worldwide, in the millions, to better understand each other.

The problem is big and complicated, and now this book has created a point of clarity to build upon. This book has the potential to advance unity in a time that desperately needs it.

This book had made the future look a little brighter.

Maarten Talbot, Producer,
Entrepreneur and Business Owner

This much-needed, unique, meticulously researched book fills a previously huge gap. Bronwyn has actively listened to and pulled together the lived experience of hundreds of people in neurodiverse relationships, giving them a powerful voice. Beautifully, perceptively written, it pulls for empathy for both partners in neurodiverse relationships in their struggle to have their needs met. Bronwyn validates the experiences of partners in neurodiverse relationships by illuminating and making explicit the negative cycles of prompting and defensiveness that are each partner's best attempts to cope with their differing attachment needs. As a therapist, it is an invaluable reminder of the cyclical nature of distress in ASC/neurotypical relationships, and how neurology underlies the coping strategies that lead to an often-distressing dynamic. Bronwyn offers these couples hope, providing constructive tips for changing the negative cycle into a thriving relationship.

Joanna Rossetti,
Psychotherapist at EFTTA

Testimonials

Relationships are always messy, and this book opens our minds to how intimate feelings, needs, and actions intersect in any relationship, including those in our own lives. As the first book in a series of three, *Have They Gone Nuts?* introduces the reader to a broad array of neurodiverse relationships between those with Autistic Spectrum Conditions (ASC) and those considered Neurotypical (NT), the ongoing interactional patterns between these partners, and the potential communication roundabout that can be formed through prompt dependency. Narratives are more than informative; they have been carefully chosen and crafted into sequenced chapters that illuminate take-home messages and learnings about challenging emotions, unmet need, self-protection, and choice making. Additionally, central concepts are supported by literature, ranging from Kanner's early observations to contemporary research findings by Attwood and others. Congrats, Bron; this book is a groundbreaker! I can't wait to read the next one.

Dr Wendi Beamish,
Adjunct Academic (Griffith University)

Dedication

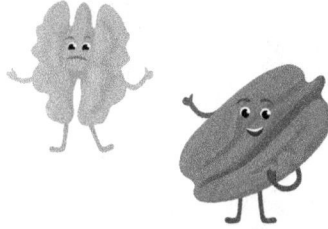

This book is dedicated to my husband Michael, who inspired me to return to further studies and continues to support and encourage me to devote time and attention to my research and writing.

I would also like to dedicate this book to my immediate and extended family members, who along with numerous friends, bestowed on me substantial understanding of the impacts of Autism Spectrum Conditions on and within relationships.

Contents

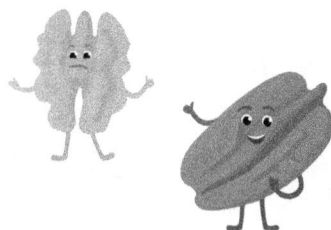

I would rather stumble a thousand times,
Attempting to reach a goal,
Than to sit in a crowd,
In my weather-proof shroud,
A shrivelled and self-satisfied soul.
I would rather be doing and daring,
All of my error-filled days,
Than watching, and waiting, and dying,
Smug in my perfect ways.
I would rather wonder and blunder,
Stumbling blindly ahead,
Than for safety's sake,
Lest I make a mistake,
Be sure, be safe, be dead.

(Author Unknown)

Foreword for
Have They Gone Nuts?

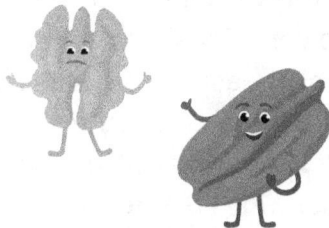

The *Diagnostic and Statistical Manual of Mental Disorders* (DSM-5-TR), published by the American Psychiatric Association in 2022, describes the essential features of autism spectrum disorder as 'a persistent impairment in reciprocal social communication and interaction' (Criterion A), and 'restricted, repetitive patterns of behaviour, interests or activities' (Criterion B). It is worthwhile exploring the diagnostic criteria in more detail to understand how the characteristics of autism will create potential challenges for an autistic person and their partner during a long-term relationship.

Criterion A has three diagnostic criteria, namely deficits in social-emotional reciprocity, reading and expressing non-verbal communication, and developing, maintaining and understanding relationships. According to DSM-5-TR, there are three levels of autism, with the signs being quite subtle for those who have ASD level 1 (formerly known as Asperger's Syndrome), in comparison to those who have a more severe and conspicuous expression of autism, namely levels 2 and 3.

The ASD level 1 deficits in social-emotional reciprocity include a lack of conversational reciprocity and impairments of the ability to share thoughts and feelings. Deficits in non-verbal communication include difficulties processing and responding to complex social cues, and mental effort and energy required to consciously calculate what is otherwise socially intuitive and easy to others. This can include a difficulty integrating eye contact, gesture, body posture, prosody and facial expressions during social communication, and difficulty maintaining effective social communication for sustained periods of time, or when under stress. There may be a preference for solitary rather than social activities, and during childhood and adolescence, a desire to establish friendships without a complete or realistic idea of what friendship entails. It is through extensive friendship experiences that we learn relationship skills, such as the art of compromise and conflict resolution, and the need for emotional as well as practical support.

Criterion B has four diagnostic criteria. The first is repetitive behaviour such as rocking which serves a self-soothing function. The second is excessive adherence to routines and patterns of behaviour which may be manifest in resistance to change, imposition of rules, and rigidity in thinking. The third is interests that are unusual in intensity or focus; and the fourth is sensory sensitivity. All four characteristics will affect a long-term relationship, in that self-soothing may be achieved by an action rather than an interpersonal experience such as affection. Resistance to change can affect the ability to achieve new perceptions and responses in the relationship. While a special interest may clearly be of benefit to the autistic person, it can sometimes be hard for their partner to appreciate this. The intensity, duration and all-absorbing enjoyment of the interest may engender criticism and conflict within the relationship, especially when it is prioritised over family or relationship commitments. Sensory sensitivity can include perceiving specific sounds, light intensity, aromas and touch at an aversive level, which may lead to trying to create an autism friendly sensory environment, in turn imposing restrictions on the partner and family.

The accompanying text for the diagnostic criteria refers to more intellectually able autistic adults learning to suppress their autistic characteristics in public and at work, and adopt a false persona to achieve social and employment success. In the early stages of the relationship, the signs of autism can also be effectively suppressed, and an effective 'mask' is created, such that a partner is unaware of the genuine degree of autism.

The DSM-5-TR text also refers to theory-of-mind deficits associated with autism, that includes difficulty seeing the world from another person's perspective. This has a significant impact on communication and conflict resolution within the relationship.

Although we have the formal diagnostic criteria for autism, I have my personal description of the condition. Autism describes someone who has discovered interests more enjoyable than socialising, and someone who has a different way of perceiving, thinking, learning, and relating; an alternative culture. These differences will gradually become apparent in a relationship, and both partners need to understand each other's 'cultural origins'.

Have They Gone Nuts? is a relationship survival guide based on the author's extensive experience and a research study that included 400 international participants, exploring how autism affects long-term relationships. It is part one of three publications and provides an overview of neurodiverse relationships. The approach is non-judgemental, describing the perspectives of both partners, and key points are illustrated by powerful quotations. The book discovers what goes on 'behind closed doors', and includes the early stages and expectations within the relationship, moving on to how specific issues start to emerge. These include aspects of communication, connection and the expression of thoughts and emotions, especially love and affection. Additional issues include meeting each other's needs and the adjustments in the relationship that may be needed for both partners to thrive or survive. A valuable and timely guide for expanding knowledge on neurodiverse relationships.

Professor Tony Atwood

Introduction

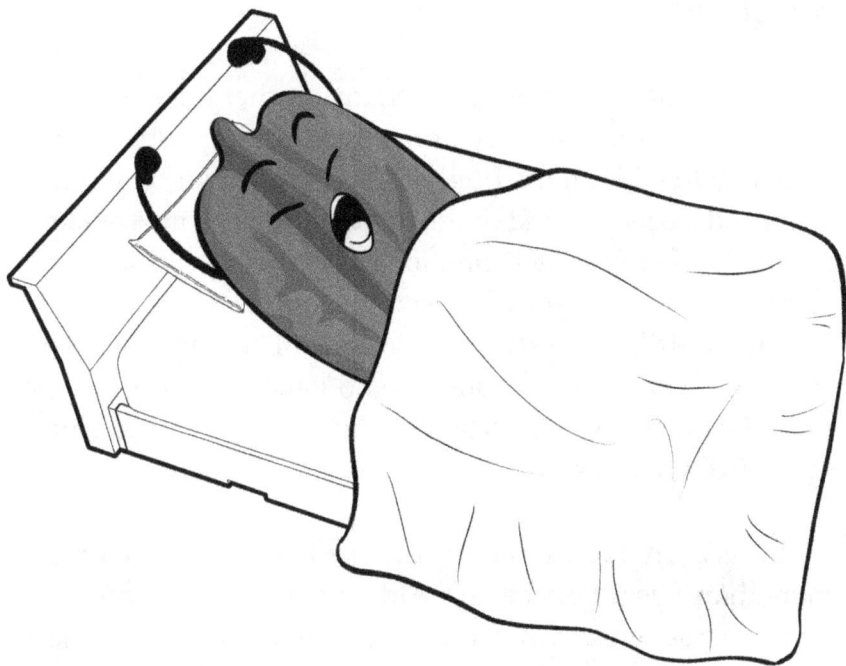

The Awakening

Have They Gone Nuts?

**'Most people do not listen with the intent to understand;
they listen with the intent to reply.'**
Stephen R. Covey,
The 7 Habits of Highly Effective People

My Story

For as long as I can remember, my mother referred to me as a bit of a 'Pollyanna' (i.e. much too trusting with a naive tendency to look on the bright side). Although a thoughtful child, of deep feeling and continuously guided by my passions, my mother found me too emotional, excessively sensitive and difficult to understand. My response was to try and hide my emotions. Still, they often engulfed me. These inconvenient emotions kept surfacing, causing emotional chaos, often at the most ill-timed moments when my mother's and my siblings' eyes were upon me.

I was born into a large family. The first of six with barely more than a year between us. Although the eldest, I grew up with a vague sense of 'not quite fitting in'. A subtle awareness that I was somehow different. While I often had long chatty conversations with friends, at home it was the opposite. They talked, I listened. Thinking through concepts deeply, they judged me as slow on the uptake, a bit simple-minded. When I did have something to say, they talked over me, interrupted me and continued with their ideas and opinions with little thought to what I might have wanted to say. I had the impression they did not want to hear much of anything from me; that they thought my conversations were about … well really not much at all. Rather than experiencing their understanding and compassion when I was distressed and in need of discussing my concerns, I endured their indifference. 'You're too needy!' When sensing another's distress and moved to tears, I experienced their ridicule. 'You're too sensitive!' They seemed unmoved by what moved me. Not that they didn't care. Merely, not affected. They did not understand me. Their contrast communicated that there was something unusual, perhaps even wrong, with me. Best to keep quiet.

Having escaped into the delight of having my own family, motherhood was a joy, a fulfilment that I had not previously experienced. However, marriage soon adopted the unwelcome childhood familiarity of indifference, ridicule and misunderstandings. Often, when attempting to compensate for being talked at and down to, not talked with, the outcome was distorted views, entangled interaction and lots of frustration. Away from my family, with friends, I enjoyed long conversations, thought-provoking exchanges and friendly banter. It baffled me. This recurring contrast remained a mystery.

Eventually, I found myself alone, and in the position of needing to provide for teenage children, with limited skills and no qualifications to speak of. It required a considerable change of direction. University life, while challenging, recharged my confidence and introduced the thought that simple-minded, I was not. A new marriage, my children now adults, and a full-time teaching career, not only provided a different way of life, but laid the groundwork that ultimately led to a discovery that I would not have found otherwise. It was this discovery that, not only revealed the answer to my mystery of lifelong contrasts, but also took me on another completely new path.

The Mystery Revealed

The day started like any other, progressing in the usual way of classrooms. I was developing an Individual Educational Plan for a child in my class, sourcing appropriate materials from the Special Education Unit, which included a checklist. An odd familiarity invaded my mind as I completed the Asperger Disorder Checklist for the child. Reminiscent of experiences past, the difficulties that this child was experiencing were known to me. An idea slowly began to emerge. Limited emotional understanding, egocentric conversations, a lack of reciprocal conversation; they were all embedded throughout the checklist. It all started to make sense. Suddenly, a light bulb when on! Many of my immediate and extended family members were most probably on the autism spectrum.

As I began to reflect on past situations with my newfound insight, I started pondering the specific teaching strategies and interactions that were required to keep students diagnosed with Autism Spectrum Conditions (ASC) engaged in classroom tasks. I had used similar tactics and procedures when attempting interactions with various family members. Discussions with other teachers revealed that these techniques were quite common when teaching students with ASC. Bryan and Gast (2000) described what I was both observing and experiencing as prompting and prompt dependency. A prompt is a stimulus used to produce behaviour (e.g. instructions, explanations and nonverbal gestures) that may not spontaneously occur (Domire & Wolfe, 2014; Milley & Machalicek, 2012). Prompting strategies are used to support students who have ASC to assist with their learning. However, when students become reliant on prompts, independent behaviour can become challenging to teach (Domire & Wolfe, 2014; Milley & Machalicek, 2012) and prompting becomes an essential requirement for them to stay on-task, complete activities and transition between activities. In a similar way, people that I knew appeared to be reliant on my prompts in my attempts to elicit reciprocal conversation, understanding and responsiveness from them. This realisation guided an ever-growing awareness that prompt dependency appeared to extend beyond the classroom. The question that surfaced was: is prompt dependency more extensive than research had indicated? A desire to know more was activated. Following my speculations, I said goodbye to teaching and started a new journey into research, ready to further explore the challenging interactions I had experienced over many years, both inside and outside the classroom environment.

One From Two

This book examines the results of two research studies. At the same time, it is also my story, and, in all probability, it is also your story. Four hundred international research participants describe the *'craziness'* and yet, also *'not craziness'* of living on the inside of a different kind of relationship: the neurodiverse relationship. A relationship that looks quite 'normal' on the outside but is anything but normal on the inside. Living in a world where other people do not understand. In a world they do not know. Where we, only we who live in it, truly understand. Only we truly know. This book opens up some of this 'craziness/not craziness'. With an unbiased approach that discusses both NT and ASC viewpoints, it gives insights and 'aha moments' that will help you navigate through this strange alternate world in which we live. It also gives others a glimpse into our world. They might just begin to understand us. Wouldn't that be a relief? For others to see what we see, know what we know, so that you no longer need to explain and explain and explain to people who still do not 'get it', no matter how much you explain. So come on a journey with me, and through the words of people just like you, just like me, our stories can be told, awareness can grow, and the understanding that we so very much deserve may begin to come our way.

So, who are these research participants? The first group were part of a Master of Special Education research, a small-scale study completed at Griffith University in Brisbane, Australia. The nine participating couples all comprised of one person who was diagnosed or self-diagnosed with Asperger's Syndrome (an Autism Spectrum Condition) and one person without ASC (considered neurotypical, or NT). The second, a larger international study, followed two years later, and was completed at Edith Cowan University in Perth, Australia, as a Doctor of Philosophy research. This time, partners, parents, adult siblings and adult children involved in neurodiverse relationships (specifically, relationships that include people with ASC and neurotypical people) were included. The majority of participants were from Australia, the United Kingdom and the United States of America, with Africa, Asia, Canada, Europe, the Middle East and New Zealand also represented. To protect anonymity, all interview participants were assigned a pseudonym.

The two studies extended over a period of eight years with the investigation of the second study based on the findings from the first. Both studies focused on adults with ASC and their close relationships, with particular attention devoted to the characteristics of prompt dependency (a behaviour that can develop due to difficulties with self-reliant behaviour and self-initiation skills), accompanied by prompting (a behaviour used to persuade, encourage or remind a person to do or say something). Confirmed in the first study, these two behaviours were found to converge into a communication cycle, caused by the very different needs of each person in these relationships to share in, or avoid, emotional reciprocal interaction. This communication cycle originated from the use of prompting, (on the part of neurotypical individuals) to gain reciprocal interaction, while prompt dependency and/ or prompt avoidance arose (on the part of those with ASC), to avoid reciprocal interaction. The second study involved comprehensive investigations into the underlying dynamics of the prompt dependency cycle and how the elements of the cycle have interacted within a complex system of competing needs, roles, expectations and problem-solving behaviours for those within these relationships.

Have They Gone Nuts? is a three-book set, designed to be an informative journey. Through the participants' narratives, we gain a unique glimpse behind the closed doors of neurodiverse relationships. Chatting and talking over many hours with the interview participants, combined with the survey data they supplied, provided such an abundance of meaningful data, that to fully share their insightful descriptions, three books were required. In this, the first book in the series, an overview of neurodiverse relationships is presented. Through the words of the participants, we begin to become acquainted with the experiences of people involved in neurodiverse relationships and why these relationships have the potential to become very different to what is considered standard for close relationships. We are also introduced to the communication cycle that can develop in these relationships, what circumstances cause this cycle to progress into a dynamic communication system and what outcomes can occur when caught in this communication system. The second book talks to clinicians and counsellors, together with family and friends, regarding the important aspects they should know about neurodiverse relationships and the communication system that can occur, in order to give appropriate support and assistance. The third talks to researchers and professionals regarding the future directions that people in neurodiverse relationships would like them to consider. The words and perspectives of both the adults on the autism spectrum, and the neurotypical adults, are interwoven together throughout the three books as we explore the different topics under investigation. Conveyed from the distinct position of each group of participants, the communication differences and difficulties experienced in neurodiverse relationships are revealed, together with the resulting impacts that each face.

The *Have They Gone Nuts?* series, is intended to be used as a resource for neurodiverse families and couples, anyone who suspects that they may be in a neurodiverse relationship, those who research neurodiverse relationships, counsellors and therapists who work with the neurodiverse population, classroom educators (due to prompt dependency's potential to be lifelong), and anyone who wants to increase their understanding of neurodiverse families and couples. It is hoped that sharing the testimonies of the 400 participants involved in the two studies will promote greater understanding of this population, and assist in bridging the knowledge gap that currently exists between many service providers and the community in general, about the unique relationship experiences of neurodiverse families and couples.

1

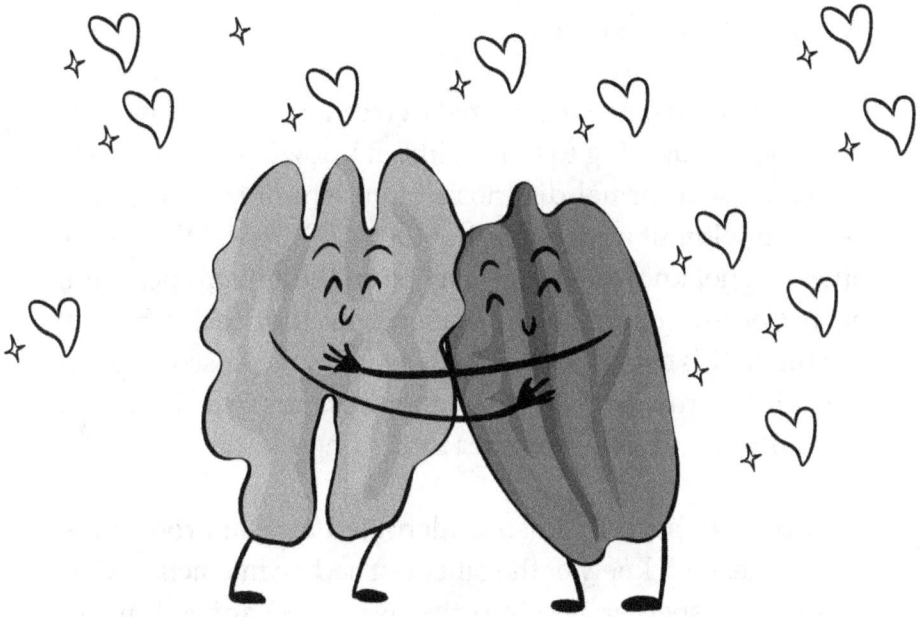

In the Beginning There Was Magic

Have They Gone Nuts?

'Each friend represents a world in us, a world possibly not born until they arrive, and it is only by this meeting that a new world is born.'

Anais Nin, *The Diary of Anaïs Nin, Vol. 1: 1931–1934*

A Regretful History

Many adults on the autism spectrum have spent much of their lives struggling to fit in without knowing why. Others, who receive a formal diagnosis of autism or self-diagnose, grew up without understanding their 'difference'. Countless others do not know that they may be on the autism spectrum, or that autism could be the reason why they feel different. Central to this overall lack of knowledge is the misconception that adults grow out of autism; that it is mostly a childhood difficulty. Yet, there is another intriguing reason.

Two men born in Austria identified autism around the same time. Both knew of the other but had no interaction. One was Hans Asperger, and the other was Leo Kanner. Kanner, a specialist in child psychiatry who had moved to the USA, identified children who were remote, unable to form bonds with people, experienced language problems and displayed patterns of behaviour, such as hand flapping and spinning (Harris, 2018). A year later, in 1944, Asperger, a psychiatrist and paediatrician in Austria, identified a more sociable group of children with less severe problems than Kanner. The English-speaking world tended to follow Kanner's reports as the definition of autism. It was not until 1981, Lorna Wing in her medical paper on Asperger's work coined the term *Asperger's Syndrome*, naming the syndrome described after Asperger. Consequently, this more sociable group became known as having Asperger's Syndrome (AS). Had Asperger's clinical account received earlier attention, the first understanding of autism may have been entirely different. This strange twist of fate was influential in the interpretations of autism. Once Asperger's work became recognised, it was realised that autism was far more extensive and complex than first thought (Attwood, 2015; Jacobs, 2006).

Although autism refers to a single syndrome, it can be understood as many different conditions, with the common factors being biological, rather than behavioural (Casanova & Casanova, 2019). Despite this, diagnosis is usually based on behaviour. Following the 2013 release of the 5th edition of the *Diagnostic and Statistical Manual of Mental Disorders*, subdivisions of autism were incorporated into a single diagnosis of autism spectrum disorder; now more commonly referred to as autism spectrum conditions. While this merging of subdivisions was an attempt to simplify knowledge and understanding about autism's complexity and streamline the diagnostic process, it has instead, created considerable disagreement, especially regarding the integration of Asperger's Syndrome[1] (Tsai, 2013). Yet, while clinical understandings of autism in children have grown a great deal since the time of Kanner and Asperger, very little has changed for adults.

---

[1] Debate continues in the autism community regarding the dissolution of the AS label within the broader classification of ASD due to the higher functioning distinction. T. Attwood (personal communication, March 17, 2015) specified that although AS is now designated as ASD level 1 (Asperger's Syndrome) in the DSM-5, the term Asperger's Syndrome is still in transition in clinical settings and within the community and continues to be applied in these settings.

The Forgotten

Keeping up with an ever-shifting understanding of autism, at any given historical moment can be challenging. However, while knowledge and understanding about autism in childhood is being regularly updated, autism in adulthood is still poorly understood (Lai & Baron-Cohen, 2015). Partly due to the obscure nature of the 'so-called' 'higher end' of the autism spectrum, and partly due to the use of social camouflaging behaviours (i.e. pretending not to be autistic), adults with AS and those with more subtle difficulties, tend not to be noticed. Often, they have been overlooked throughout their school life and into adulthood, since they look and talk 'normally', even if not quite 'fitting in'. The subtlety of AS is also sometimes its curse (Stoddart, 2004). An 'appearance of normal' means that, even though they themselves, and others, have a vague understanding that there is some difference, there is often a general lack of understanding by both parties as to exactly why they feel different, and why they are treated differently (Portway & Johnson, 2003, 2005; Stoddart, 2004).

Since research continues to focus heavily on children, few people understand how autism manifests in adults. Many adults have remained undiagnosed and unrecognised throughout their entire life. Behaviours, such as repetitive body movements, have been often mistaken for signs of obsessive-compulsive disorder or even psychosis. Mental health professionals often lack the skills or experience to distinguish autism in adults, from diagnosed disorders with which they are more familiar (Lehnhardt et al., 2013). Tantam (2012) points out that 'the ASDs are conditions in which there is no sharp distinction between normality and pathology'

(p. 179), and as a result, the contrasts, the inconsistencies, and the assorted characteristics that are unique to each individual, make it extremely difficult to identify different, yet overlapping aspects of the spectrum conditions. To further complicate matters, although each person on the autism spectrum shares similar difficulties, the degree, extent and quantity of these difficulties influences how well, or not so well, any person adapts, functions, and interacts with others. Is it any wonder that misunderstandings, confusion and even falsehoods abound? Coming to terms with autism's range of functioning ability that varies in combination and severity, between and within individuals (Akshoomoff et al., 2002) is a challenge. As a result, adults with ASC have largely been overlooked by the public, healthcare providers, researchers, academics and policy makers, and the needs of autistic adults, the needs of their significant others and their specific family needs have been neglected. The aim of this series of books is to go some way towards addressing this oversight.

The overview of autism's historical foundations presented above supplies the backdrop to the studies that are reported in these books. A prevalence study of the Centres for Disease Control early in 2022 confirmed that the majority (59%) of autistic individuals do not have an intellectual disability. These books are directed toward those who do not have an accompanying intellectual disability; to discuss the experiences of people involved in neurodiverse relationships, to provide insight into specific obstacles that may be encountered and to illuminate how some have found a positive way forward. While most of the participants involved in these studies discuss their romantic neurodiverse relationships, some also discuss their neurodiverse relationships with adult children, parents and siblings. So, let's meet the participants.

A Short-Lived Magic

At the start of a relationship, an adult on the spectrum is often described as someone who is kind and attentive, someone who is intelligent and often gifted in areas of maths, science, technology, medicine, art and music, and someone who is usually very truthful (Mendes, 2015; Moreno et al., 2012). There may be a noticeable 'quirkiness', or an almost childlike or innocent quality, which often adds to their appeal. Many also have high-status occupations, including engineers, computer specialists and academics, constantly showing extraordinary competencies at work. Many participants report that the beginning of their relationship was quite amazing. When interviewed, Sophie (NT) had not long started a new relationship. She described the early stages:

> *He is more genuine and honest than most men I have dated or been in a relationship with. I love how he is clear and honest and doesn't play emotional games like my ex-husband of 16 years did.*

Yet a common feature to autism is an average to high intellectual capacity that is accompanied by a lower than usual social capacity (Baez & Ibanez, 2014; Deisinger, 2011). Compensating for their lower than usual social capacity, Attwood (2015) describes how some adults with an ASC can approach finding a prospective partner much like finding a job; that they formulate a mental 'job description' and search for a suitable applicant who can compensate for their particular difficulties in life. 'Once a candidate has been found that person is pursued with a determination that can be hard to resist' (p. 317). Dana (NT) shared how that was the case for her:

In the Beginning There Was Magic

I remember when I first met Miles, he seemed very driven for us to have an ongoing relationship. I was less so, and he really worked on me, and I settled for it. I agreed to it, and we wound up raising a family and I did not really feel like I was part of that relationship even though I was there.

Using their intellect, adults on the spectrum can become quite resourceful at masking their differences (Pearson & Rose, 2021), leading to high proficiency in abilities to conceal many of their eccentricities until well after a romantic relationship has developed. Richard (ASC) explained the reasoning behind this behaviour:

... Prince Charming and Snow White, they get together, they have the big wedding and go off into the sunset and you don't see the rest of their life together. I suppose that's how we get information ... on whether you're suitable for marriage and things like that, but the actual day in, day out married life and what's normal you can't. Even if you bought a book off the shelf that only applies to the person who wrote the book and you're pretty much learning things as you go along.

Yet as a relationship develops, this lower social ability begins to surface. A higher intellect cannot compensate, and quite quickly, the early attentive and devoted stage of the relationship is brought to an end. Attwood (2015) confirms that 'the courtship may not provide an indication of the problems that can develop later in the relationship' (p. 318). Therefore, it is only after some time when the first bloom of courtship fades that their inadequacies mostly become clear. Lucy (NT) described this 'before and after' sequence that often occurs over the course of a developing relationship:

In the first eight months he was so affectionate, and of course listening to Tony Attwood speak a couple of years ago, it all made sense, that they go into character and once they've got you, they don't need to do that anymore. So ... he would just turn me around and give me a hug and a kiss ... Later on ... I said to him 'Before you used to, you have never done it since'. He said, 'Well that's then. This is now.' So that's how cold he could become ... He's got me, so he doesn't need to act any more.

Diana (NT) expressed a similar view, sharing some of the changes that had occurred as their relationship had progressed:

Before we were married, he'd probably ring 10 times a day. We were talking all the time ... but often these days there can be really awkward silences. This morning he's come in from mowing the lawn and well the whipper snipper has disappeared ... and instead of being able to just have a normal conversation ... he had to just sit and think, being in his own thoughts ... I said to him 'You've got a lot of the rest of the day you can be by yourself and be in your own thoughts about it, is there any reason why we can't have a conversation or enjoy some time together while we're having coffee?' But that was really difficult for him, just little things like that in everyday life ... communication is not there. Half the time seems like he's on a different page or planet.

Sally (NT) echoed this sentiment, highlighting the communication disconnect that only seemed to appear after some time:

When we first got together, we met online, and we both worked at different places and we did a lot of emailing and

*then once we got together, he used to email me every day
'Morning sweetie. How's things going?' … I wanted it to
carry on and he just stopped. And I had to say to him 'I want
you to write to me, it doesn't matter whether its meaningless
to you, it means something to me, and I want you to send me
the morning emails.' But when he moved in, and we were
together it sort of gradually petered off.*

Similarly, Rae (NT) described how her husband disengaged
from her only after her relationship had progressed:

*Before we got married, he used to come round to my house
and he would be there to one o'clock in the morning every
night, and then when we got married it was like … a bird in
a cage, once they get you, they just leave you alone. 'Okay,
I've got her now. She is in the cage. I can go back, go on with
what I was doing before.'*

Richard (ASC) confirmed his demonstrations of affection to
his wife had lessened over time:

*At one time she … said 'Are you having an affair?' … and I
said 'No, there's nobody else and I do love you, but I suppose
… I'm just not showing you as much affection as what I
did 20 years ago.'*

In Summary

A diagnosis of autism in adulthood, while gradually
increasing, is still relatively rare. Accordingly, many
adults fly under the radar while at the same time feeling
obliged to pretend not to be autistic (Mandy, 2019). This

'pretending to be normal' is a very common social coping strategy used by most adults with ASC (Hull et al., 2017). Although it has its purposes, for example to achieve goals, such as getting an education, holding down a job or establishing relationships (Mandy, 2019), the drawback is that others who are observing the camouflaging behaviour can believe that the person is quite different. In that case, they are getting to know someone else and not the authentic person.

Given that first impressions of the communication abilities of those with ASC are usually inaccurate (Aston, 2003), many relationships begin very differently to how they continue. It is only after a relationship progresses that the differences become clearer when difficulties begin to surface. Most NT participants discussed this matter, describing their first impressions of their partners and the disappointment that they felt when realising their impressions where not accurate. However, ASC participants mostly gave explanations for their actions. They did not appear to consider the false impressions that camouflaging behaviour may present to others.

The next chapter explores more fully how this camouflaging behaviour impacts on each as a relationship progresses. We delve into what happens when the real person behind the mask is revealed, what happens when both are confronted with a reality different than first anticipated and what they felt as a result.

2

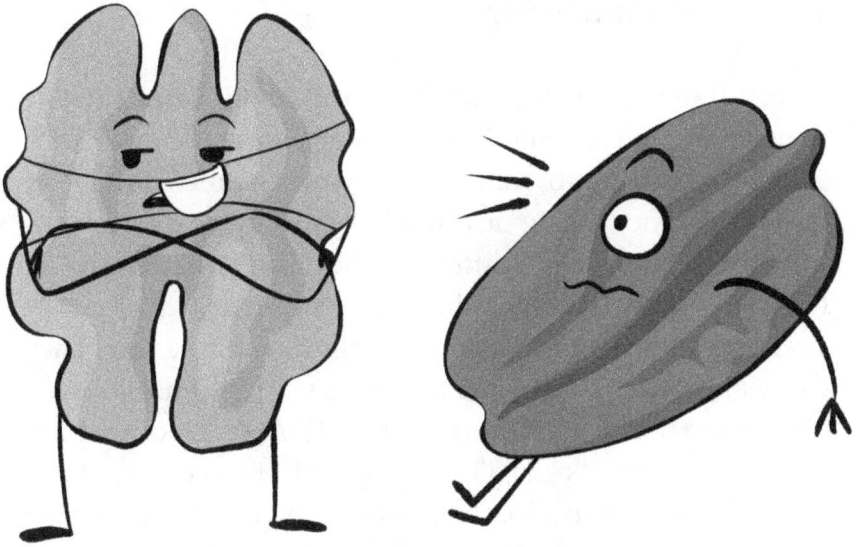

The Mask
Begins to Fall

Have They Gone Nuts?

**'You trade in your reality for a role.
You give up your ability to feel,
and in exchange, put on a mask.'**
Jim Morrison

The Art of Camouflage

Just like a chameleon, most of us want to blend into our respective environments. Usually, people do not want to 'stick out like a sore thumb', for to do so can sometimes mean they are in for some teasing or ridicule. Naturally, people on the autism spectrum are no different. They also want to blend in. They want to do similar things, act in similar ways, and be just like everyone else in their neighbourhood or setting. They also want to form relationships and have children. However, from when they are young, people with ASC notice they are different to their peers. They observe their peers 'reading' social situations and instinctively 'knowing' how to react to other's thoughts, feelings and intentions, effortlessly and accurately (Arioli et al., 2018). They notice that their peers can figure out how to easily form and keep friendships. These abilities are elusive to an autistic child. Wanting and trying to connect and engage with their peers, their social approaches to other children are usually awkward and often rejected. They regularly experience teasing, ridicule and bullying for being different. Yet, they are different. They do not blend in socially. They do tend to 'stick out' in social settings. That is because their brain wiring is quite different to the typical brain. A study by Sato et al. (2017) showed that grey matter volume in those on the autism spectrum was lower in the regions of the brain that process social signals, when compared to the neurotypical participants in their study. They suggested that this difference was partly responsible for the widespread 'social brain' network differences in ASC.

Another difference is a distinctive tendency to see and seek patterns and systems. While typical brains do this too, the autistic brain is particularly skilled in this area. Due to the negative responses they received from their peers, to compensate, people with autism are often driven to the sidelines to quietly observe the play, and the social interactions, of others. With the intention of studying and imitating, they become proficient at watching and learning the patterns, absorbing all that they see. Like an actor learning lines, once they have acquired a 'script' they use their script to perform a role and successfully blend into their environment. They start to do as others are doing, they start to talk like others are talking and by suppressing their autistic behaviours, they appear just like everyone else. Thus, they blend in. They appear neurotypical (Lehnhardt et al., 2013; Livingston et al., 2019). This process is described as masking, camouflaging or creating an alternative persona.

Interviews revealed very different consequences of this camouflaging behaviour between the two groups of participants. While camouflaging usually triggered a sense of normalcy and predictability for ASC participants, for NT participants it caused a disconnect between their private and public life. Samuel (ASC) described the sense of normalcy that his pretending everything was 'normal' gave to him:

I can't provide her with what she needs in the relationship because of my Asperger's … We have the kids' girlfriends' parents over at night and we just act like any other normal couple. Dinner is made. We sit down and drink wine and chat. I get to have a family … So, we're getting things from it. It's just not your standard relationship that's all. So yeah, we just get on with it, we've got our friends, no-one really says anything, they just come and visit, and we act like a couple and it's all good, yeah.

However, Rae (NT) described how her husband's 'alternative persona' caused a rift between her private and her public life:

People say, 'But what do you argue about?' Because in public Isaac seems, such you know 'Mr Congeniality' … Everybody just thinks he is so lovely. Everybody just loves Isaac … He's the perfect gentleman and he's not nasty and of course when other people see him, he's jovial … when they see him socially, they say 'everybody loves Isaac' … 'What do you fight about?' and I thought, 'I can't even begin to tell you. I can't even put it into words because that sort of interaction doesn't happen when you are out socially.'

Similarly, Haley (NT) discussed the differences between her husband's public and private behaviour towards her:

In public … it was what was socially acceptable, so he would always come and put his arm around me, and I used to think, 'Well you can't any other time, but you come and make out that we are really close' … When we were in public, he would make a big effort like it was important because 'this is my wife sort of thing'. It was all about … the image, it's all about what is perceived to be the right thing.

However, Rachelle (ASC) expressed her irritation at feeling required to camouflage her autism:

The Mask Begins to Fall

I feel like I'm faking it every day and I can't be the person I want to be … I just have to conform to what society wants me to be and I can't talk to people the way I want to talk to people. I have to put in all these nice words and use inflection in my voice and try and act normal … People think I'm rude … and I'm just surrounded by people who aren't on the spectrum, at work and with my husband … It's like being from another planet, speaking another language and yeah, it's difficult. It's like I wake up every day and when I leave the house I have to put on a mask and pretend … when we see other people communicating and smiling at each other and chatting away … the small talk, it's all fake like it's all just nothing, meaningless, we don't find any meaning in it … it looks meaningless.

Usually, camouflaging is used as a temporary remedy for autism, useful for specific purposes, such as to do well at work or to achieve a long-term relationship. Therefore, when a relationship has been formalised, the mask is allowed to fall, and a greater expression of autism is seen at home. Georgia (NT) shared her views on seeing the person behind the mask as the reality of autism became apparent to her:

You shouldn't have to tell a 54-year-old man of three children, in the head of department, 'If the trash can is full, take the damn trash can outside.' It's not a natural and healthy way, I don't think for a man and a wife to be, and that was one of the things that I discussed with my counsellor, is that if we were to continue as man and wife, how would it impact me having to tell this man how to live … a man who is capable of running a department, being the head of people, is obviously incredibly bright, manages multi-million-dollar grants, but at home, is basically a child. When at work … they are functioning, they

*take initiative they get stuff done, but when they come home
... they can't do anything, you have to call them, or you have
to initiate it, or you have to tell them what to do ... I couldn't
reconcile that. I cannot tell this man what to do at home, like
you end up being their mother.*

Since camouflaging is an adaptive mechanism used to
achieve certain outcomes, it may not be as conspicuous to
co-workers as to those at home and may produce a different
result at work than at home. Wally (ASC) discussed these
work/home differences:

*I function well at work ... Work is the place where you
know your place, you know your structure, you know your
boundaries. There are limitations to the subjects that are
discussed ... In your workplace you're there because you
know your shit in that area, but in a family all rules are off
... I think I've done the right thing, said the right thing but
I can't understand, I can't clearly understand the effect.*

Yet, every so often, away from the home environment, the
mask may slip, and other people also get to see behind the
mask. Holly (NT) described this situation:

*One of my friends, she said to me not long ago ... 'When
Jack's with you and we come to your place for dinner I think
he's absolutely normal' but ... 'I took him to the pub the
other night ... I realised when he's away from you, he's not
normal.' So, this friend could see that when Jack's alone it's
kind of like the smoke screen has gone.*

A Masquerade Malfunction

Due to a gap between intellectual ability and everyday functioning ability (Attwood, 2015), people with ASC are prone to anxiety, especially when required to join in with social interaction (Dubin, 2009; McVey, 2019). Many find the know-how involved in beginning and continuing a conversation particularly difficult. Not knowing what to say, or when to say it, often leads to attempts to conceal a lack of skill with scripts and pretence, or too much talk, or not enough talk, or the wrong type of talk. Camouflaging behaviour and 'pretending to be normal' however, is emotionally and cognitively exhausting. Alongside this, people on the spectrum may experience an ever-present dread of making mistakes. The awareness of the existence of social rules, the desire to conform to them, but an awareness that they don't completely understand them and don't entirely 'fit in' understandably causes high levels of anxiety. Additionally, the desire to have a relationship, but struggling to carry out the ongoing daily necessities of relating, can further increase the stress and anxiety levels. Over time, this stress may contribute to feelings of low self-worth and depression. Being disconnected from the authentic self, camouflaging behaviour can become a vicious circle of increasing anxiety, which in turn, increases the camouflaging behaviour to overcome anxiety.

In addition, many people with ASC often have a low motivation to change any resulting unhealthy patterns of behaviour due to the desire for sameness, a core feature of autism. Comfort can be gained from a fixed routine or set of behaviours. Rules and routines promote a feeling of safety and being more in control of the environment. When developing a pattern of behaviour that suits a particular purpose, such as bringing anxiety down, this behaviour can become set in stone. Fully unchangeable.

A realisation of autism can also lead to an unwillingness to change. A study on loneliness and depression by Han et al. (2019) found that, in the general population, suffering depression was a frequent trigger to experiencing anhedonia (i.e. loss of pleasure). However, the exact opposite took place for people with ASC. Both social and non-social anhedonia, or a loss of pleasure, was found to be associated with a knowledge of autism symptoms, which set in motion the development of depression. So, for the general population depression leads to a loss of pleasure, but for the autistic population, a loss of pleasure leads to depression. The study by Han et al. (2019) found that when an adult with ASC had a better understanding of conventional relationships and of social communication, they were more likely to perceive their behaviour as atypical or 'strange', and this knowledge was found to lead to depression. Symptoms of depression can also impair social functioning (Zimmerman et al., 2018), which in turn can expand relational problems. When involved in a relationship, these circumstances may contribute to a low motivation to engage in, contribute to, and persevere with, the ongoing interaction necessary to sustain relationship health.

Multiple instances of malfunctioning interaction can add to an unwillingness to change unhealthy patterns of behaviour due to the constant social communication difficulties that people with autism experience. A fear of interaction failure can follow. Why change if it is going to be wrong anyway? A fear of failure can produce a cautious, evasive approach to interaction, leading to feeling helpless and furthering the stress and anxiety felt in conversations. Learned helplessness is a behaviour that can occur due to negative attitudes that have developed over time in reaction to past failures, resulting in conceding defeat. It came through strongly in the studies that a fear of failure in conversations, triggered by anxiety, caused ASC participants to use avoidance behaviours. By withdrawing they were trying to keep control of a conversation in a situation where they felt overwhelmed, out of control, and in fear of failing. Interviews also revealed that while both ASC and NT participants experienced similar feelings of stress and anxiety when speaking with each other, the explanations for the feelings were very different.

For participants with ASC, a fear of failure, the complexities of emotional conversation, and multiple experiences of malfunctioned communications were reported to be the main motivations behind their feelings of anxiety, stress and a sense of powerlessness. Many ASC interviewees discussed these anxieties. Wally divulged that his fear of getting it wrong overshadowed his desire to try:

I don't know how to … initiate. I certainly don't know how to ask for that … it's partly probably the fear that if I ask for it and it's not given or that I'm asking and it's the wrong time and I'm talking about verbal or physical … if I've misread that it's an inappropriate time and it's brushed off then I won't know whether it's for now or forever …

Rachelle's desire to talk was diminished by her anxieties:

Talking to others definitely brings on a level of anxiety and stress and it's just incredibly uncomfortable. I only want to talk to people when I need something out of them.

Have They Gone Nuts?

Mareena's anxiety dominated her actions:

> *With great anxiety, I'm treading on eggshells because it seems that anything I say, is going to be taken the wrong way and used as a basis for further judgement.*

William explained that fear of failure was due to his anxiety:

> *Well, if it's just doing things, there's a certain amount of fear about failing to do it properly ... But if there's other people involved, there's even more fear involved about interaction with other people. I've got to overcome that all the time.*

Ronald shared how anxiety caused him to withdraw into himself:

> *Isolation, I just isolate. I can hear words being said and ... I just close down. It just doesn't come in ... I do hear the words, but I don't actually hear, you know, I hear what's going on, it is just a lot of words. I don't sort of, pick them up to deal with them, they are just noise.*

Wally lamented the fear that caused him to adopt a cautious, evasive approach to interpersonal interactions:

> *It's a scary place to go ... so I will avoid ... it's avoiding that confrontation ... and then she says, 'You'll go silent for a couple of hours and then ... you'll talk about stuff like as if nothing has happened.' ... and I'm like 'Well what else am I supposed to do?'*

Whereas Mark confided that anxiety tended to make him dependent on seeking more attention from his NT partner:

I tend to suffer from a separation anxiety, so if Kay is ignoring me or does not want to interact with me, for whatever reason, it does cause me some angst, and I will try and interact with her some way, communicate with her but, that can also be the source of conflict. If she's busy doing something and I need her attention for, even the most trivial reason, it's something I try and push, or have done in the past, but it is something I need to learn to back off from. It is just one of those traits that … needs to be altered.

Although NT participants also reported feelings of anxiety, it was for very different reasons. The avoidance behaviours of their partner/family members, together with an inability to progress through conversations caused their anxious feelings. Ryan shared how he tiptoed around difficult subjects with Rachelle:

Well … broaching subjects, I know we don't agree, she is not going to change her mind that readily … so it does make it fraught in terms of broaching subjects, knowing that it is most likely going to be an ugly outcome from it, and that we will be at loggerheads, and I have to walk away. Ah, she will walk away sometimes herself too, to be fair, and it doesn't make getting engaged in a topic, easy … I feel my tension levels rising walking through the door at home whereas at work I was calm and happy and, and it should be the opposite way around, but often it is not. I am a lot happier at work in many ways than at home.

While most NT participants understood that their partner/family members experienced anxiety when conversing, they felt the absence of conversations, deeply. Katy, Ronald's wife, discussed the impact of Ronald's anxiety on her:

He is, in his home life, he is very anxious. Highly, highly anxious person. Gets very aggressive verbally. I don't have any fears about him physically, but verbally he gets very aggressive, very loud, and that is fairly frequent.

Katy also gave an explanation as to why she thought people with ASC may be so avoidant:

I just can't believe that it is anything but 'this is going to cause a lot of emotional upheaval, I am going to remove myself from it' … So I think, as an adult, an Aspie adult may be, is deliberately shutting down that episode in order to comfort themselves.

Daniel (ASC) conveyed the sentiment of both groups:

There are subtle but radical differences in our world views. There are things about being autistic, and being not, that defy communication.

In Summary

Although, social camouflaging may offer some advantages for adults on the spectrum, more often than not, it creates additional problems, both for themselves and for others. It can hide an individual's difficulties, preventing them from being understood and helped, yet a greater concern is that the pretence can lead to the development of mental health challenges (Mandy, 2019). Additionally, it blocks others from getting to know their authentic selves.

When added to the distinguishing features of communication that are characteristic of autism, camouflaging behaviour presents multiple problems for relationships. The core problem for people on the autism spectrum is difficulty with social communication, especially figuring out the nuances of affectionate interaction. The conundrum is that, often they have proficient levels of language. Their aptitude to use language skilfully can work alongside difficulties with social communication and a failure to process the language of others. In these studies, the participants revealed that unseen turmoil behind closed doors was triggered by the mask coming off at home but staying on in most other situations. When accompanied by the day-to-day reality of living with high skills in certain areas coupled with low skills in others, a disconnect between the public and private lives occurred that led to an unmanageable, hidden reality within the confines of the home. These fundamental features of autism are central to understanding how the majority of problems tend to remain behind closed doors, leaving those in neurodiverse relationships in an unseen but complex and baffling position. As a result of the mask going back on when leaving the house, the mayhem remains hidden within the home.

Triggered by the social and emotional conversational difficulties that are inherent in autism, the next chapter looks inside the home and delves into the extensive interaction problems that usually occurs in neurodiverse relationships. The participants discussed at length their attempts to find a way through their differences. The ability to convey affection, express feelings and emotions, converse about personal matters, and participate in deep and meaningful conversations, alongside occasional experiences of alexithymia, were particular areas of difference which caused these relationships to develop very differently to a conventional relationship.

3

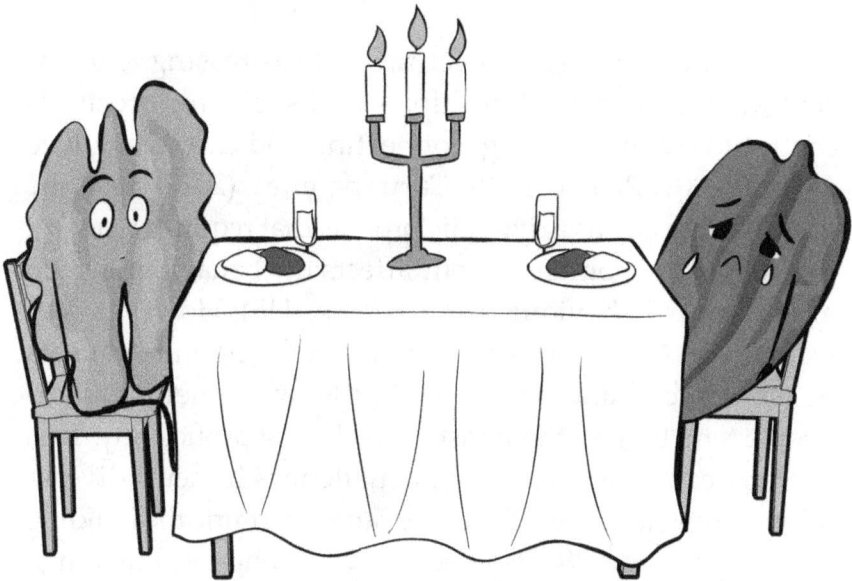

The Language of Affection

Have They Gone Nuts?

'When dealing with people, remember you are not dealing with creatures of logic, but creatures of emotion.'

Dale Carnegie

Affection's Anguish

Communicating, connecting and expressing love are central to healthy relationships – and social reciprocity is central to communicating, connecting and expressing love (Aston, 2001; Rearn, 2010). Caruana et al. (2017) describe social reciprocity as a dynamic process that requires working together since 'your behaviour affects my behaviour, which affects your behaviour in return' (p. 115). However, key features of ASC include marked and lifelong impairments in these social and emotional skills, while neurotypical people tend to have them instinctively and proficiently. This contrast can create substantial challenges in neurodiverse relationships, as these differences can undermine the building of intimacy and closeness necessary for long-term relating.

Additionally, deep and lasting emotional connection comes from the choice to consistently put effort into understanding and decoding the expectations and needs of the other, through the commitment to share in social reciprocity. When successful, this allows a person to feel connected and affirmed. It conveys the message of caring in a deep and personal way. It increases relational security and satisfaction. It fosters health and wellbeing. It safeguards against stress, depression and anxiety. Therefore, connection is both influenced by and strengthened by cultivating social reciprocity. In view of the fact that relationships are transactional, both the giving and the receiving have associated health benefits (Garris & Weber, 2018). In other words, the social and emotional support gained from emotionally connected relationships sustains each individual and the relationship (Burleson, 2003; 2009).

Interaction differences between the two groups of participants were found to create incompatibilities in emotional interaction and connection needs. The main contributing factor for a lack of affectionate and meaningful conversations within neurodiverse relationships was that ASC participants frequently averted social reciprocity by avoiding opportunities to express feelings and emotions, to converse about personal matters or to take part in deep and meaningful conversations. In contrast, NT participants needed to experience frequent expressions of feelings and emotions, frequent conversations about personal matters and frequent deep and meaningful conversations in their relationships. These opposing differences caused an inescapable and persistent gulf that opened between the different needs of the two groups of people.

The Alexithymia Affect

Alexithymia is described as a pronounced difficulty in identifying emotions, describing one's own emotions, and also communicating about emotions (Wilkinson, 2016). According to Milosavljevic et al. (2016) alexithymia is a personality trait that has frequently been found in autistic people and has been linked to impairments in emotion recognition and empathy. Griffin et al. (2016) explain that 'alexithymia is a word derived from ancient Greek and literally translates into *without words for emotion*' (p. 773). Alexithymia is associated with an outwardly-faced way of thinking which involves four cognitive and affective dimensions: difficulty identifying and describing subjective feelings; difficulty distinguishing between feelings and the bodily sensations of emotional arousal; restricted imaginative capacities and a shortage of fantasies and dreams; and an externally oriented cognitive style (Eid & Boucher, 2012). When an individual with autism also has alexithymia, it can present as an added difficulty to the meaningful conversation needed for relationship health, especially with the requirement of giving and receiving emotional language within close relationships.

Feelings and Emotions

Expressing feelings and emotions were very different experiences for the two groups of participants. It was something to be avoided at all costs for ASC participants, while for NT participants, expressing feelings and emotions was a source of enjoyment, a process that resulted in closeness, and a welcome practice to be embraced as much as was possible.

Most ASC participants explained that expressing their feelings and emotions was challenging for them. Although recognising that their partner/family members wanted more from them, the challenges that they faced meant that their preference was to avoid these types of conversations. Demonstrating features of alexithymia, Wally described the difficulty that trying to express feelings caused:

> I express it by saying I don't want to talk about this because I'll get upset … Trying to identify what the feeling is and how to deal with it is really hard and it gets in the way of rationality.

The Language of Affection

Similarly, Rachelle explained how limiting emotional conversations functioned well for her, while also acknowledging that Ryan was not satisfied:

> *Well, it meets my needs, I'm happy just to have … even just a 10-minute conversation a day and that forms for me a good marriage, but he wants more constant connection throughout the day. He doesn't feel satisfied.*

As a result of sharing how connection, interaction and the intimate sharing through communication were simply not a priority for him, William was inadvertently conveying the message that he chose not to put effort into understanding and decoding the expectations and needs of others:

> *But as an NT, you seem to appreciate the social interaction where I couldn't care less. I just do it because you're expected to, you have to. It's just an interruption and an annoyance.*

Mary questioned why it was even necessary to interact and communicate affection, stating that she preferred inanimate objects for that reason:

> *Like I don't understand why people tell each other that they love each other all the time. You say it once and that's what you mean. If the parameters don't change then why do you need to say it again, because you have already told them … I love my carefully contact-wrapped, beautifully preserved … book collection as much as I love people. It is the same kind of love … and it sometimes is easier to love the inanimate because I don't have to interact.*

Have They Gone Nuts?

Most ASC participants reported that anxiety, confusion and intensity of emotion caused them to avoid emotional conversation:

MALCOLM   *She will say 'Oh Honey, tell me how you are feeling.' And of course, to me as an Aspie, I have got nothing to talk to you about. Just like saying, 'Can you speak some Russian to me?' And I will say 'Honey, I can't answer that. I have got nothing to say to you.' Like I will talk spontaneously, if planet Malcolm is in the right position, but that is it, and of course, she finds that challenging.*

SAMUEL   *It would be far too intense for me to cope with ... so mostly, no I don't really want emotional discussions because things usually end up causing a fight and usually end up escalating.*

TOM   *I prefer to keep to myself or talk about topics that are interesting to me. Emotive conversations make me feel anxious.*

While most NT participants confirmed they were aware of the difficulties that their partner/family members experienced with expressing emotions, it did not defuse their disappointment that the lack of these types of conversation meant limited meaningful interaction and connectedness for them. Winnie described how conversations became 'stilted' when focused on emotions:

The Language of Affection

Sharing of emotions is not something that we do very often or with a great deal of depth ... if I ask him how he is feeling he won't respond to those sorts of questions ... he cannot express how he is feeling and similarly if I express how I am feeling his understanding is very limited ... so that makes our conversations quite stilted around emotions.

Similarly, Maggie shared how her son's difficulty with expressing emotions affected their relationship:

I find that there is a lot of work on my part to manage the relationship. My son tends to really lack empathy ... I expect a little bit more loving care the way I give to him and I never ever get it, so I've learned to just not expect that thing from him ... I know he feels love ... but he doesn't know how to integrate the expected expressions of love into a normal kind of interaction with people.

Ruth shared how uncomfortable her husband was with expressing his emotions; however, the unintended consequence was that she did not get to experience his emotional expressions or build their relationship together:

I would not describe my husband as warm or affectionate ... Displays of affection or any declarations of love or affection are foreign and make him feel uncomfortable ... Most of our conversations are exchanges of information.

Most NT participants felt a deep discontentment about their partner/family members' predisposition for detached, unemotional interacting. They needed more affectionate and expressive forms of interaction. They needed reciprocated positive emotional encounters. Left without these types of conversations, the resulting lack of understanding, lack of responsiveness and lack of emotional connectedness left them feeling insecure and rejected. Many revealed that the pursuit for emotional connection became a string of failures. Instead of continuing to strive for what they could not achieve, many decided that the next best thing was to drop these types of conversations themselves. Wanda expressed the widely held position within the NT group:

> *I try to not express too much emotion in what I might say, so in conversations if I think that I'm not being understood these days, I tend to just back out of the conversation.*

Most NT participants also lamented the absence of closeness with their significant other, and what the resulting lack of affection meant to them:

TRACY   *When I get close to him to express my emotions and my love, he is not ready to receive or to accept me, as if he is rejecting me. I asked him not to remain like an ice cube, without acknowledging my presence, when I approach him.*

NORA   *I can't need stuff emotionally from him and if I do it has to be like I can't be emotional about it ... but I think the bottom line is just move on, just get over it.*

RONDA   *The closer I would try to get the more he would run away ... [it seems] talking with me is not desirable; being around me is not desirable.*

Comments from the survey showed similar difficulties and attitudes toward emotive conversations between the males and females within each group of participants. A female ASC respondent said:

I have great difficulty communicating my emotional state.

A male ASC respondent reported:

I find it hard to process/think about, relationship/feelings stuff.

In contrast, a female NT respondent expressed:

[I] have to be more rational and not emotive at all. As soon as any emotion is involved, he shuts down.

A male NT respondent said:

It's become second-nature, now, to avoid emotional responses and getting angry ... everything will escalate, and the situation will be dreadful for many days. It's better to remain factual and emotionally neutral. I deliberately don't think a lot about how much emotional warmth I would like in our relationship, because it's not going to happen ... Why torment myself? It's better to get on with life and learn how to make it work as best we can.

Personal Matters

The difficulties those with ASC had in expressing feelings and emotions influenced most of their personal interaction within their relationships. Many participants reported that the meanings behind a great deal of personal interaction were regularly misunderstood by both parties. The frequent response, for those with ASC, was to avoid getting into personal conversations altogether. The NT participants reported that the only time they experienced these types of difficulties themselves, was when conversing with their ASC partner/family members. These challenges created considerable issues for both parties within their relationships.

Generally, ASC participants felt that participating in personal conversations was a frustrating and undesirable task, made even the more difficult by complications with communicating meaning. Edith explained her process:

> I actually have to talk it through and then I understand what it is … the thinking and the feeling are separate.

Jim described his frustrations while revealing his lack of understanding and lack of working together with Dianne:

> Can't even get my point across, so that's … why I try to keep to the facts because you can't argue about facts … I wouldn't be able to get my explanation out quick enough or out enough so that she would understand … a fruitless exercise … She just feels that I'm not trying, but the point is, 'what are you supposed to be trying at?' … I'm really good at doing things, but when it comes to emotional or communicative, no, I'm ratshit.

On the other hand, Mary described the confusion that was caused between her and her partner Alex, due to her inability to understand herself:

The Language of Affection

There have been times where things have been so incredibly easy, and then other times really difficult to nut out, and I think a lot of that has to do with the way I convey things. Some things are just a lot easier for me to convey than others ... Alex can only act on the information that I give him and if I don't know it myself, and I'm behaving in a way that Alex is going 'You are saying this, but you are behaving like that. Do you really understand what you are dealing with?' And I will go 'I've got no f**king clue ... I don't know what I am doing or feeling.'

Most NT participants also felt that personal conversations became an often-frustrating task. However, for them, it was the laborious and confusing patterns of conversation that often occurred within their relationship that made conversing problematic. Their attempts to consistently put effort into understanding and decoding the expectations and needs of their partner/family members, often resulted in intended meanings becoming muddled for both parties. Sally explained how difficult it was to get her meaning across to Samuel, her ASC partner:

I can't tell him what I'm trying to tell him, because he won't listen and ... it's really hard to get him to focus on what I'm actually trying to say, and what's important to me ... what I am actually trying to get across, and trying to explain tends to get completely lost in all the words missing, and the exaggerating, and the going off on tangents, and he interrupts me all the time ... so I don't feel heard.

Grace described how she thought Malcolm heard her through 'an Aspie filter' and as a result, he did not fully understand her:

It is really challenging for both parties, but I suppose the most challenging, from my perspective, to communicate to an Aspie, is that they are always going to interpret you through an Aspie filter. You can never get away from that, and even when they are [in a] productive, open, resourceful happy state to receive your information, they are still hearing it through that filter and that's the challenge.

She expressed how she had tried to come to terms with it:

I think that, to me, that is the biggest challenge that he, they will never get what you truly mean. They will get aspects of it, but they'll never really get that and you've got to be okay with that. As long as they get the gist of it … He is never going to hear what I meant. Even if he was totally receptive, you know.

Meaningfully Deep

The differences in need for emotional conversation and an inability to strengthen connectedness through successful social reciprocity resulted in a distinct lack of deep, meaningful conversations within these relationships. Not only did those with ASC report a preference for more objective, logical types of conversation, but some conveyed dissatisfaction with the necessity of also having to participate within meaningful conversations. Wally shared that he understood the importance of meaningful conversations, and then revealed the reasons that he avoided them:

I have an intellectual belief that it's important to be able to have that deep exchange of ideas and … a respect that other people's feelings are different, and I understand that that's a necessity so … of course it would be better to do this, but it's a scary place to go … so I will avoid.

Similarly, while recognising its importance, Tom disclosed his dislike of meaningful conversation:

I recognise the necessity of having meaningful conversations if I want a close connection. However, I do not like this type of conversation.

On the other hand, Sharon named the features that formulated meaningful conversation for her:

Warm and affectionate conversations in my context translate into deep and meaningful intellectual discourse that may or may not involve our feelings for each other.

Alternatively, Barry illustrated a vague understanding that there was no connection between him and Hope and that something was missing, but he did not appear to understand that deep and meaningful conversations were needed to build the connection that he knew was missing:

Where I see there is no connection … well why is that connection missing? Why though? I don't know. So, there is something I am missing, and I have to go about it mechanically and if someone said, 'Look you have got to go do this, this, this and this,' I can go do that. I can go through the motions. But still, I would have to be going through the motions and she would pick it up. And a lot of times if I have tried to do that, it gets to a certain point where eventually she goes, 'Oh this is back to square one again.'

Generally, NT participants lamented the lack of deep, meaningful conversation that they required for emotional connectedness. The result was feelings of dissatisfaction. Tracy shared what she had put in the survey and why:

> *I answered in the questionnaire that I was never satisfied with our emotional connection now, simply because there is none.*

Then she expressed how the absence of deep, meaningful conversation within her relationship affected her:

> *James does not understand what I am after. He doesn't know why I would not feel 'close' to him … I have just stopped trying to have deep and meaningful conversations with him … I end up having those conversations with other people, friends, or my children.*

Likewise, Sabrina shared a similar sentiment, labelling her relationship as a business relationship:

> *There's just no more affection left. It's truly a business relationship … It's just day-to-day things that anybody would deal with but there's no emotion, there's just none.*

Beth described the complexity of trying to hold important conversations that were impeded by Christopher's perseverative comments:

> *He can get onto the one topic and just go on and on and on and I'll have to change the subject, I'll have to say, 'Now look I've got to discuss this with you, it's really important.'*

The Language of Affection

While Ruth said that her husband's conversations were deep, they were not deep in the way that she would like:

> *I feel like he has the ability to have a deep conversation. It's not emotionally deep though; it's intellectually deep.*

Nora said that she wanted to be in the same boat as her partner:

> *So mostly, I wished for a deeper emotional connection, I wished that we would be in the same boat together and experience things together and reflect things back off each other, but on an emotional level, we don't ... that's not how we roll together. The way we operate is that we are vastly different in how we process things and look at things ... and we both like to talk about certain stuff ... but it can't happen emotionally which is why I mostly want more ... Yeah, it's hard.*

However, she lamented that he did not want to be in the same boat with her:

> *He's like 'We're just journeying through life together on our boats.' I'm like 'What do you mean boats?' He's like, 'You know, you're in your boat, I'm in my boat' ... So for him it's not like 'we're in the boat together'.*

Comments from the survey illustrated these differences too. Although he understood the necessity of having deeper conversations, an ASC survey respondent shared how he struggled to accomplish it:

Communicating about internal feelings is difficult for me, and I often have difficulty responding to questions in deeper conversations. Don't understand myself and my desires in order to share them. I don't think I 'get' relationships and personal intimacy – may know the theory but struggle to apply it ... Only in the past five years have I understood that I have an ASD – but in hindsight can see relationship difficulties throughout our marriage that it has impacted and exacerbated.

An NT survey respondent shared her perspective on the point that the ASC survey respondent had raised in his survey:

I have explained to my partner that the way I feel connected to him is through talking and that it is hard for me to maintain a feeling of connectedness when he barely responds. He made more effort for a while but seems to have given up, perhaps it is too hard. I try cognitively to value all the actions he does which show me he cares because he does do lots of nice things for me, but somehow, they don't mean as much to me as a conversation. I have to deliberately think about the things he does and place value on them, there is not the automatic satisfaction that comes with a meaningful conversation.

In Summary

The giving and receiving of social, emotional and affectionate interaction are critical components of most close relationships, however major shortfalls in these areas are common in neurodiverse relationships (Lewis, 2017). Most close relationships demand a certain amount of dexterity in the giving of and receiving of affectionate and emotional interaction, together with adequate involvements in interpersonal and conversational interaction and acceptable understanding of social norms. However, typical relational qualities are challenging for adults with ASC to achieve, which produces a very different form of relationship to the conventional.

Both sets of participants talked at length about the difficulties that adults on the spectrum experience when required to take part in social and emotional conversations and reflected on the resulting lack of affection and connection within their relationship. However, it was found that this produced very different outcomes for each group. The ASC participants discussed how their differences and difficulties led them to avoid expressing feelings and emotions, conversing about personal matters and partaking in deep meaningful conversations. They reported that they were fine with less than the usual amounts of all things social, particularly all the emotional aspects of relating.

On the other hand, NT participants usually do not experience the same social interaction difficulties commonly faced by those on the autism spectrum. They reported that they were not content with the minimal amounts that their ASC partners and family members were prepared to provide. Likewise, they also wanted to be able to give more to their ASC partners and family members. They wanted more reciprocity, not less. The very different emotional connectedness needs resulted in incompatibilities between the two groups of people. These incompatibilities are discussed in the next chapter.

4

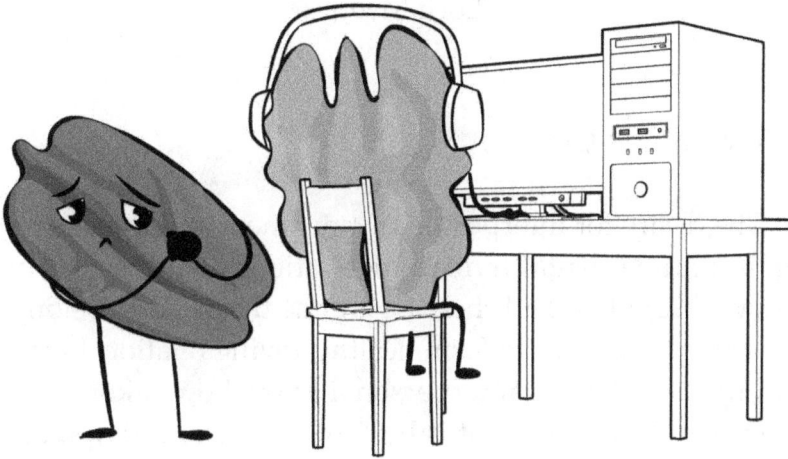

A Collision of Needs

**'Needs cause motivation.
Deep-rooted desires for esteem, affection,
belonging, achievement, self-actualisation,
power and control
motivate us to push for what we want
and need in our lives.'**
Lorii Myers

When Needs Collide

The desire for interpersonal attachment and to be cared for, are fundamental human motivations. Baumeister and Leary (1995) identified these desires as the 'need to belong'. However, the ability to form healthy, loving relationships is not innate. Effective interpersonal know-how takes much practice over a lifetime. It is built over time and developed during reciprocal interaction with others, through a strong motivation to belong to others. This interaction is critical to achieving meaningful connected relationships with others and to negotiate the multitude of differences that springs from everyone's distinct temperament, specific belief system and varying childhood experiences.

People who are NT, usually experience a sense of wellbeing when their need to belong is fulfilled by frequent, productive and deep social encounters. The opportunity to communicate, connect, express love, and give and receive emotional support through reciprocity is a fundamental part of interpersonal interaction for them. In contrast, people with ASC experience difficulties with communication, social interaction, and processing their own and other people's emotions. With an in-built self-bias, together with an innate preference for more non-social experiences (Benning et al., 2016), naturally, they focus less on others and place less emphasis on social encounters and related emotional connectedness (Gillespie-Smith et al., 2018). Therefore, the deep social encounters, the emotional connection, the giving and receiving emotional support that are required to fulfill a need to belong for individuals who are NT, are not sought by those with ASC. This extensive difference has the potential to cause difficulties in some relationships.

These differences were reported by participants with ASC to be the main influencing factors in their avoidance of conversations. The desire ASC participants had to avoid most interpersonal communications was seen to be the catalyst to each group of participants experiencing and assessing their relationship in very different ways. The desire to avoid, as opposed to the desire to engage in interpersonal communications caused an imbalance in affection and connection needs.

Most interviewees with ASC reported that they noticed their partner/family members' need for expressions of affection, however, they confirmed that they did not have the same need:

WALLY   *Well we don't have the kind of rituals that I observe in others … We've been married nearly 30 years and we've never had the things that other people express … we've never been, for example, in the habit of a kiss goodbye on the way out in the morning, even the 'Honey I'm home' is a stereotype which doesn't apply. It's just never been something that we do.*

Have They Gone Nuts?

SANDRA   *I do know that he wishes that we would be more affectionate with each other and … I guess I don't have that feeling as much.*

ANDREW   *Like we had one guy stay with us … Couldn't do without his wife for one second and so he was on the mobile to her the whole time. 'How are the kids? I want to hear them and get the kids to say hi' … I don't have that type of relationship with Hazel, cause if I went away for a month, I would go 'Fine, bye.' … Cause she's been away for three months overseas. I would just go 'Fine.' I go about my business and when she is back, I go and fetch her at the airport and say 'Hi' … She will go 'Did you miss me?' and I will go 'Oh, yeah.' But not intensely. Cause I know that she is okay over there. I know she would phone me if there was a problem, and I would phone her if there was a problem. And that's it … So it is funny like that and so that's the main difference I have seen people that I know well. How their tie is with their wife … they have a big attachment where they can't do without their wife … Funny I wouldn't do that.*

Most NT participants realised that a difference in need for affectionate and deep meaningful conversations was the cause of much discord. Regardless of the friction, they needed what they needed, and lamented the lack of these types of conversations within their relationships:

A Collision of Needs

RYAN   *I feel that she does enough in a sense to try to satisfy my needs emotionally, she certainly tries. I do give her some leeway knowing that she does have an issue in terms of empathy around the whole ASD stuff ... She has to kind of write things out, think things out, and try and work out ... what a neurotypical would probably just automatically intuitively understand and do or expect.*

QUINN   *It's kind of hard for my husband to connect with me emotionally so I think whatever I do ... like hugging him or telling him I love him is enough for him. He can't do the same for me. It doesn't matter if I tell him this is what I need, however many times, he doesn't seem to be able to get to the level that I need him to be.*

TRACY   *But with time, I stopped trying to have deep conversations with James because I went away empty each time ... In the end, you try to protect yourself from constant disappointment.*

MAGGIE   *Whenever I want to talk about anything that's emotional, he will either shut down or just change the subject ... I'm closer to some of my friends, I have better communication with my friends ... but I have my daughter, I have my husband, there's a chance that my son-in-law has, and there's a chance that my grandson has, so [I'm] surround[ed by] AS.*

The Great Escape

People with ASC often have difficulty with pragmatic language (i.e. the use of appropriate communication in social situations by knowing what to say, how to say it and when to say it) (Patton, 2019). Difficulties with expressing their wants and needs can result. When misunderstanding others, or others misunderstanding them, they may not always offer clarification or seek clarification. These types of language difficulties, combined with emotional language difficulties, and difficulties with giving and receiving of affection, were the main triggers to the avoidance of and/or disengagement from interaction with their partner/family members. Three central avoidance behaviours were found: a desire for company but without any emotional conversation, a desire for times of solitude to relieve tensions, and a desire to take refuge from social activities through undertaking special interests. These behaviours were the processes through which most ASC participants endeavoured to meet their need of interaction avoidance.

Company Without Expressive and Deep Conversations

While avoidance of emotional conversation was found to be the main driving force for escaping most forms of communication, it was confirmed that the motivation was not because of any lack of love or caring for their NT partner/ family members. Instead, ASC participants revealed their love and affection in other ways. They expressed that they did experience contentment in the company of their partner/ family members, and often wanted to spend time with them, but they did not want to take part in the emotional aspects of conversations. Placing less emphasis on social encounters, being together was enough for them. Doing things, rather than offering emotional support, was their preferred way to show affection. To decrease the likelihood of emotional conversations, they often withdrew from the company of their partner/family members. They highlighted that this lack of involvement was not from a lack of love for the people within their close relationships, rather, it was their anxiety about participating in emotional conversations, together with a lack of an equal need to deeply connect through conversation, which caused this behaviour:

> MURRAY *I think she's secure in the fact that ... the amount of affection isn't based on the amount of love.*

> WALLY *I don't feel like we have to be conversing, interacting, whatever, all the time. I just want to be in the same house ... and just be in the same space and ... not feel like we had to have frivolous conversation. Just be around each other ... at home and weekends because you know I have a full week and I'm buggered. I need that chill out space at the weekend and she accepts that, she knows that, and she also likes to just sit around and read a book sometimes too, but we can go for hours and feel like we're going to have to talk about something.*

> SHARON *I expressed my affection through daily small acts like waking earlier to make coffee and breakfast for him before he went to work*

> *... as a form of affectionate support and to relieve his work stress so that he was a happier person ... I was unquestionably a 'wise' advisor and somewhat 'dutiful' wife. I think my partner perceived my role and position as more functional than affectionate.*

RACHELLE *I'm kind of just okay with the level that we've got now. If I wanted to have fixed it, I would have increased the level of conversation or intimacy up to this point, like this is the level I'm happy with ... I don't think he is happy at all.*

Meanwhile, this withdrawal behaviour left NT participants in distress. Most shared that they understood that their partner/ family members with ASC did not have the same need for emotional connection, and that anxiety was a frequent cause. However, most felt that the lack of emotional conversations, unresponsiveness to their emotional conversations, and the resulting lack of emotional connectedness, were the most difficult things to deal with in their relationships. A few described how they tried to adjust. Others lamented the lack of emotional support:

SABRINA *I'm the one who's dissatisfied. He's kind of okay because he's getting whatever limited needs that he has met.*

SHIRLEY *I thought I was the sort of person that did require that ... before I got into a relationship with Jill but Jill doesn't give those freely so I've kind of learnt not to place too much*

> *expectation on that … over the years I've lowered my expectations.*

TRACY   *I don't think he tries to connect in any way now, other than through acts … One day he cleaned out the inside of the dishwasher … and said to me: 'You must be so happy to have a husband like me! There's not many men would do this, you know!' … I just stood there speechless … Like I ever cared a hoot about the inside of the dishwasher!*

MAGGIE   *There was no affection, there was no encouragement, there was no hugs, unless you know you've just been chastised … then you start to say, 'Well am I really worth anything?' and living with that is really hard to find an identity for yourself, and self-esteem, yeah and self-confidence, that's what I battle with all the time.*

Solitude to Relieve Tensions

It is well known that adults with ASC have a higher need to seek solitude with lower levels of need for social interaction, when compared to NT adults. Interviews confirmed that tensions felt from all forms of personal and emotional conversations, together with a need to think problems though alone, rather than talk them through, were contributing factors for adults with ASC to seek regular amounts of seclusion. They shared that they often preferred to spend time alone than with their partners and family, sometimes just to relax, sometimes to recover from tense conversations or interaction difficulties, and sometimes to gain relief from resulting social interaction anxieties. Many described how connection, interaction and sharing through communication, were simply not a priority. Their preference for non-social activities however, meant spending time alone was a regular priority:

> STELLA   *Our communication was better before we had a child and while I was in work, partly because we spent less time together ... I feel I would be happiest to spend my days reading and listening to music, without him and our child, and that doesn't improve relationships ... sometimes I just need to be left alone and it would be the greatest way of showing he cares.*

> SAMUEL   *Her personality is drawn entirely to the world of people, absolutely, and if it's not to do with a person and what they're doing, it simply does not exist to her. She will not notice anything else around her, anything to do with the garden, unless I tell her to go out and have a look at it, anything that I find interesting is really of a vague interest to her, simply because it's not to do with people, whereas people are part of my life but it's only a fraction of my world, whereas it's her whole world.*

> RACHELLE *I'm quite happy to sit in silence ... what's going on in my own head is far more important than what is coming out of other people's mouths.*

A Collision of Needs

SANDRA   *If he's trying to maybe be emotional or affectionate with me and I'm doing something else, it gets that kind of anxious feeling of having to stop what I'm in the middle of and put my focus on what he wants, because in my mind I'm like, 'I'm in the middle of something, I have to finish this and I'm enjoying what I'm doing', so I don't want to stop and do something else.*

While a few NT participants described their attempts to accommodate their partner/family members' need for solitude by looking to other sources of connection, the main outcome for them was a loss of the desired interpersonal connection within their relationship:

TRACY   *Although the emotional connection, even though I felt it was sometimes present in the earlier stages of our marriage, just never lasted more than a few days. The emotional connection I craved seemed to drain my husband, seemed to wear him out, seemed to demand all his energy, so that he had nothing left to give after a few days.*

LUCY   *I know they like their solitude, I know you've got to give them their solitude and I don't have an issue with that because I've got a good social life, I've got good friends.*

QUINN   *I just express how I feel and he either chooses to respond or not but ... that's just the way they go ... He would shut down and not say*

61

anything and then I just mainly cry because I'm a very sensitive person and it frustrates me … He doesn't talk. I have to fill up the silence, so I just keep talking … He shuts me down. Gotta do something to cope with it.

GEORGIA   *He … said to me 'A touch from you or a warm kind gesture and everything would just fall away … everything would be okay', so … for him it was like minimum amounts of affection whereas for me it was like, 'No you need more to do than that.'*

Refuge in Special Interests

Both ASC and NT participants mentioned how those with ASC experienced high levels of anxiety when involved in emotional and social conversation. While it was the main reason for them to avoid communicating, the systematic conversation avoidance that they performed, such as shutting down and withdrawing or melting down and exploding within their relationships was problematic for the health of the relationship. The interviews confirmed that a focus on special interests usually gave ASC participants a way out, to either, avoid emotional conversation when possible, or to achieve emotional recovery after going through an emotional discussion. A greater focus on special interests was an enjoyable way reduce their anxieties. Many ASC participants recognised that time spent on a special interest impinged on family time, however, this awareness did not often translate into changing their single-mindedness. Instead, a preference for solitude or separate activities

A Collision of Needs

led them to customise family time to accommodate their special interest. When conversation became personal Stella described that:

> *I often feel as if I'm on trial, that I don't know what to say, that my brain becomes paralysed and frozen.*

Whereas Sandra expressed how difficult it was for her to put aside her interests for the sake of others:

> *Yeah, I do see that getting very focused and engrossed on something, and then if something else needs to be done ... I get more anxious about having to leave what I'm doing to mind what they need.*

What emerged from the interviews was that the entire group of participants with ASC often felt more dedicated to their special interest than to their relationships. Their self-bias caused their significant others to become a lower priority:

> RACHELLE *Yes, I'd certainly want to spend a lot more time on my interests than I do on family time and I have to be mindful that my son won't be young forever and what he remembers now will be his memory of his mother when he was young and I have to try and relate to him and my husband and not just be pulled into my interests.*

> SAMUEL *I discovered photography ... and it became my obsession and unfortunately I get most of the pleasure for my life from that, and she doesn't share that ... That's probably led to*

> *where we are now because I cannot give up*
> *what I love, she is unable to join me in it and*
> *therefore we've agreed to disagree on that, she*
> *does her thing and I do mine.*

DANIEL   *Yes, my tendency to spend hours absorbed in*
computer games, books and other distractions
does not pass without comment. Cathy's
distress motivates me to stir though, and we
find peaceful equilibrium again.

TERRY   *If I'm in the zone or flow with something I'm*
actually doing that's visual and tactile my
hearing shuts down ... so when Kim is trying
to talk to me about something I've zoned out.

Murray's perspective revealed that he considered finding a constructive way to confront the matter:

> *I think ... the Asperger person can be quite obsessive about*
> *things so part of what we work with is 'Okay, you're naturally*
> *obsessive.' ... I used to gamble ... and that was time away*
> *from the family and not a positive thing to be doing, whereas*
> *now I cycle and go in bike races every weekend ... once I*
> *understood Asperger's like that I'd say 'Okay, I'm obsessive,*
> *I need to find something positive to be obsessive about, not*
> *something negative' ... me spending time away to be fit is*
> *... a very different attitude from her versus me spending*
> *time away to gamble.*

NT participants reported feeling quite differently about their partner/family members' special interests. Despite having some understanding of the need for a special interest, many NT participants felt that the devotion given to it, rather than to them, was a major difficulty in their relationship. The frequent result was feelings of resentment as they felt they had to compete with the special interest for time and attention. Most revealed that the affection and attention that they looked for from their partner/family members was left wanting:

RUTH   *Yes, my husband used to spend substantial amounts of time on special interests or hobbies … It was horrible … He felt that he was doing important things and 'having experiences' and that was really hard for me. I felt like I didn't matter, and he didn't want to spend time with our son.*

NORA   *You can't compete with a special interest … we were having major fights before the whole AS thing came on board … because the special interest somehow is them figuring out who they are, creating a self. I really feel that my husband, like his self-esteem and his self-identity is being constructed through the output of this special interest and how that's measured in the marketplace.*

SABRINA   *So he just spends hours in the evening watching these bike races … He doesn't get it, it takes time away from every part of our relationship, his daughter's relationship.*

DAWN   *I have had to learn to be very independent. Hobbies! … When he starts a new hobby, oh my God, the world moves for that hobby … and*

> *that has been a thing throughout our marriage
> … he plays computer games … I think it is just
> daft to sit and play golf on a computer when
> there is a golf course out there … so yes there
> has been a lot of times where whatever is the
> latest interest has been absorbed to him to the
> distraction, to the dismissal of everything else
> in our lives, me included.*

RENEE   *I've always felt that I've never been No.1 in
> Patrick's life … so I've always come second
> to other things and the other things have
> included his mates early on when we were
> young, his job, his job and his job, and then
> latterly his kind of obsession with saving and
> that is: saving power, saving money, saving
> resources … so all those things are ultra-ultra-
> important to him, whereas little old wifey here,
> and little old kiddies here, have never been that
> important.*

The Great Debate

As a rule, adults who are NT experience very little, if
any, verbal and non-verbal language problems. They can use
their emotional and interpersonal communication skills to
build a closely connected relationship. Consequently, when
involved in a neurodiverse relationship, the considerable
quantities of pleasurable social and emotional interaction
they desired was found wanting. Their competency with,
and need for, reciprocated expressive and deep conversations;
reciprocated affective companionship; and reciprocated

affective conversational intimacy were also found wanting. Instead, they mostly experienced minimal amounts of affectionate interaction, insignificant amounts of warmth and passion, insignificant connectedness and considerable amounts of impersonal and superficial conversation. The result was a relationship that that was unsatisfactory for them.

Reciprocated Expressive and Deep Conversations

While both NT and ASC participants were mostly in agreement with each other regarding the need for meaningful conversation, it was found that agreement did not translate to attainment of reciprocal meaningful communication between them:

Georgia (NT) stated:

That's the problem with that reciprocal relationship that most of us in this type of relationship are searching for, but an Asperger person doesn't seem to be able to give or understand.

Terry's (ASC) statement revealed that he could not apply his understanding to his relationship:

Kim would like to have more communication interaction with me … rather than just sit and listen.

A lack of the reciprocated expressive and deep conversations that NT participants were seeking within their relationships, was one of the main reasons that the emotional connectedness that they were also seeking, did not develop. While they understood that their partner/family members did not often perform well and/or want to engage with these types of conversation, they nevertheless wanted their partner/family members to understand that they had a necessity for these types of interactions to feel cared for, wanted and emotionally fulfilled. They reported that the support that they gave their partner/family members, to encourage more of the positive emotional encounters that they wanted, was often thwarted by a lack of engagement with their efforts. A frequent result was that superficial conversations became the rule:

WINNIE   *Our day-to-day conversations are superficial. They revolve around chores and how your day has been and it will be very concrete answers like, 'I did x, I ate y for lunch' ... so there's no exploration of in-relationship interaction ... It's the realisation that ... things are not going to change, therefore my wanting more affection is only going to make me unhappy ... so my response is to go and do more things with other people.*

RENEE   *I feel that my husband has no idea of me as a person. He struggles very much with understanding anything to do with me as a person, so he sees me as a physical person, obviously, but really you scratch the surface, and he doesn't know me at all ... Conversations tend to be for example 'How did you go at work today?' 'Oh okay.' 'Did you see so and so today?' 'Oh yeah.' 'How are you feeling today?' 'Okay.' ... See what I mean? Superficial.*

A Collision of Needs

HOLLY   *If we were to talk about anything very, very*
          superficial. For example, the weather, what
          the traffic is like he will volunteer that stuff
          but if we were to have to talk about the fact
          that one of the children was having difficulties
          with work ... it would always be instigated by
          me.

Another result was that their own commitment to the relationship was altered by the absence of deep and meaningful types of conversations:

TRACY   *Reactions and lack of reaction also set up*
          barriers which kill emotional reciprocity. If,
          when you speak to someone, the person does
          and says nothing, one gradually stops speaking
          to that person, so: no emotional connection. If
          he regularly says things which hurt you, you
          progressively pull back emotionally and get
          your emotional input elsewhere.

WANDA   *I've kind of given up ... I think I've kind of*
          worn myself out ... I've sort of reached that
          point of not being hurt anymore and trying
          not to expect anything and I don't have the
          answers.

NORA   *Well obviously we've both got different*
          emotional needs and I probably have a higher
          need for emotional sort of intimacy and
          responsivity and desire to sort of be seen by
          my partner. He's happy with how things are
          because he doesn't need as much on that scale

and basically there's a disparity there which
means I'm lumped with how it is.

They also thought that their interactional dealings and experiences were not representative of what would be considered 'normal' for close relationships. For example, Dianne summarised the general NT sentiment:

I actually sit on the train and look at couples that sit together on the train and converse with one another and think 'Gee, I wish my relationship was like that.' ... Nothing is kind of natural if you like. Nothing comes because it's fun. There is no fun in the relationship. It is always tentative. Jim is always very defensive ... there is no spontaneity. There is no ... hug as you walk in the door ... or a bit of fun, or a bit of laughter. Not even normal conversation ... Jim will tell me three days later something that's happened, and yet we will sit at the dinner table just about every night with nothing to say ... and the couple will sit and just even the way they look at one another. You think, 'Oh wouldn't that be nice if he just looked at you one day like you are the best thing since sliced bread.' ... probably that's what I miss the most. The natural things that I would see as naturally occurring, you know, in a relationship.

However, many ASC participants described how difficult it was for them to communicate in the way that their NT partners/family members wanted. Most realised that this difficulty did lead to complications within their relationships. Some did not. A realisation, however, did not transfer to understanding just what these complications entailed, how they were involved personally within the complications, or how much impact these complications had on their partner/ family member. Subsequently, many had little idea of how to do things differently. In view of that, there were many ineffective ways of dealing with the absence of conversations that their partners/family members wanted, including the claim that difficulty with communication was more an issue of the listener rather than the speaker.

Dianne's husband, Jim (ASC) highlighted how he thought that Dianne was responsible for the communication troubles within their relationship. He shared the opinion that Dianne was not as responsive toward him as he thought she should be. At the same time, he illustrated that he lacked the awareness that it was his unresponsiveness toward her regarding his need to be 'more communicative'. Therefore, he missed the point that being 'more communicative' did not just mean an expression of his feelings, but that he also needed to listen and respond to his partner's emotional needs. Thus, illustrating his lack of awareness that communication was intended to be with his partner; about her, and her feelings, as well as 'his feelings':

'But Jim you've got to be a bit more communicative.' Okay if you haven't got someone who wants to listen to you, how can you be more communicative, and also express your feelings? Huh, feelings okay, yeah, I feel sad, I feel alone now, I feel angry, I feel upset. The issue is the partner says 'get over it' so how do you, how do you do it? Give me a pill ... It's probably just my partner. Like I'm sorry, but I'm no good at interacting with people outside my work environment. Is that a crime? Is that something that I should be ashamed of? I don't think so, but the point is just give me a tablet, or if this is the way that you got to do it, just say okay, this is the way you've got to do it. I will follow orders. To turn around and say, 'Well you've got to be a bit more considerate, a bit more passionate'. Oh yeah right okay.

Have They Gone Nuts?

Like Jim, many participants with ASC mentioned that they did not perform well and/or want to engage with reciprocal affectionate and meaningful conversation. Some commented that they were often not aware when their significant others required reciprocal interaction and/or connection from them. Some reported that they did not know how to respond even if aware, while others mentioned that sometimes they became annoyed by their partner/family members' efforts to get them to reciprocate in conversations:

RICHARD   *But reading somebody's emotional signs … the light bulb doesn't go off in my head.*

SHARON   *There were times that my blunt way of expressing my feelings resulted in unpleasant outcomes as he felt hurt … even though to me, it was just what I feel. Personally, I didn't feel that I should be too careful with my words with my partner, or to have to sugar-coat it, as they were the real feelings. Constructively, I felt that we should be working on why I felt what I felt, instead of focusing on the words I used.*

SANDRA   *He generally wants to figure things out to the end. It really bothers him when I try to just end it and move on. If I'm just like there's nothing else to say and I start to walk out of the room, or if I just turn over in bed and want to go to sleep … he's told me it really bothers him, so I try not to do that much, but if it's in the moment I'm not always caring … I just want to go do something else and end that situation.*

However, Max reported that even though it was difficult for him, he recognised the importance of working at reciprocal interaction and/or connection for the sake of the relationship:

> *So, it's got to be by invitation in much the same way that any change in a relationship is really by invitation, I invite you to meet my needs and to come into my world in a way that's really helpful to me and without that kind of reciprocal meeting of invitations you know the relationship does in fact suffer because it doesn't change, and the needs aren't met.*

Reciprocated Affective Companionship

For NT participants, the concept of 'companionship' included warmth and closeness with opportunities to experience deep, meaningful conversations and to discuss important, personal and relational issues. Although ASC participants said that they understood logically the importance of these forms of conversation within relationships, the idea of 'companionship', for them, included much less conversation, merely being in the same space, or harmonious individual activities. Since the ASC concept of 'companionship' did not require consent, it was possible to be achieved. However, the NT concept of 'companionship' required agreement, therefore it was more difficult to achieve.

Most NT participants reported that the lack of companionship led to fragmentation of their relationship for them. Some described how they became resigned to a connection deficit, while others described the sadness that caused them to turn away and try to gain companionship outside of their relationship. A few tried to appreciate the difficulties and accept the situation. It became clear from the interviews that the entire group of NT participants felt disconnected from their partner/family member in some way. The absence of the close companionship that they were looking for with their relationships, but were unable to remedy, gave rise to mixed feelings including discontentment and frustration:

QUINN   *I would ask something … and he would never respond so sometimes I would go to bed crying, I would cry myself to sleep he never came and held me, he never came to ask what was wrong … I can't get over the hurt of some of the things that have happened, I'm not sure how to get past that and he can't connect with me emotionally to give me the assurance that I need … so I need to get over it on my own and I have no idea how to do that.*

LAURA   *He does not seem to want or solicit greater connection except that he does sometimes seem to seek out my presence … I wish he paid me more attention, noticed me more, shared more of his inner life with me … [I] often feel we just live two parallel lives.*

Maggie expressed her pain that she could not connect with her daughter:

It's just a nightmare and I battle with the lack of connection, especially with Chloe I battle with being able to hug her … that sensory stuff … and I get that … I will live with the pain of that, but if I could have more of an emotional connection with her that would be fine.

A Collision of Needs

Grace (NT) described the challenges she faced with her husband, Malcolm. However, she reported that she was resigned to try to come to terms with the situation:

> So … something's come up, and in a normal relationship, as soon as it comes up, you blurt it out, you don't really think about it. You go 'This has bothered me' or 'that' … and you've picked a time where it is just so inappropriate. Not for a 'normal' person, but so inappropriate for someone who has Asperger's or autism … I had to really deal with that need to have, I suppose in a sense, to be heard … I really want to be able to say, 'This is how I'm feeling about it', but I know I can't in that moment … sometimes it will be two or three days till I feel he is receptive.

Malcolm (ASC) shared his point of view about Grace's attempts to connect with him. Interestingly, he referred to NT individuals as 'humans'. He had also explained that he had given his 'Aspie moments' a name, calling it a 'Matilda'. He shared that this name was to help minimise the difficulties his differences formed:

> Very challenging … basically humans want to talk, Aspies don't want to hear, or what they interpret is completely different to what they are hearing. How do you get past that? … Even in my Aspie moments, when I am in my cupboard sulking, having a Matilda moment, I am processing. Processing what happened, why am I in here? How can I make it better? I don't want to do this again. You know, and even when I am doing it I am thinking 'Oh God why am I treating Grace this way?' Like, just ridiculous. I haven't talked to her for two days. And I process that, and it takes time. Sometimes I just can't get out of that. It goes around

and around in my head. But as time has gone on, I have learned, you know I can stop it, sometimes, almost instantly. I will have a Matilda, and an Aspie moment and then ... 'No, there is a better way to do this.'

Unlike Malcolm, Samuel (ASC) reported that he did not appreciate the requirement placed on him to talk and connect to Sally's satisfaction:

I felt Sally used talking as a weapon almost as it would drive me nuts, it would be far too intense for me to cope with ... and she would insist on continuing the conversation until it drove me nuts.

Sally (NT) expressed sadness at that:

So, affection wise it's yeah, I have to completely look elsewhere for that sort of support so it's very sad but again it doesn't faze him ... I mean I guess I wish that he cared.

Other ASC participants doubted their conversational abilities:

RICHARD   *Some people can ... just go up and start talking to anybody about anything ... Denise says 'I wish you would talk more' but ... sometimes I think what I have to say is boring or uninteresting or I don't know.*

TERRY   *I suppose that's probably about one in 10 that we manage to talk things through to Kim's satisfaction.*

A Collision of Needs

Still others strove to achieve some form of connection, but often found it too difficult:

> WALLY   *If I can't control that outpouring then you can't actually have the conversation. You can't actually explore the meaning because I'm so overwhelmed by the emotion of it, that rationality becomes very difficult ... I call it avoiding ... that confrontation. It's not avoiding a confrontation with her, it's avoiding a confrontation with me ... So, I'm aware of Alexithymia, I'm definitely an Autistic person who also is alexithymic and trying to identify what the feeling is and how to deal with it is really hard and it gets in the way of rationality. It gets in the way of progress in that, yes it's a tough place to go and although I want to go there, I recognise the need to go there, it f**ks me up.*

> RACHELLE *It's like we just go through our daily lives, and we don't actually stop and connect much.*

An anonymous NT survey respondent revealed the frustration of a lack of emotional connection:

> *My experience of the relationship would be better if I felt connected ... and received acknowledgements that we exist as a couple. Communication is almost always frustrating.*

In contrast, a survey respondent with ASC confirmed that he did not have the same need for connection that his wife did:

I have great difficulty meeting my wife's needs and find it difficult to change my patterns of behaviour and conversation. I don't feel the need to connect emotionally in the way she does.

Reciprocated Affective Conversational Intimacy

Clearly, less than satisfying relationships are experienced when difficulties in emotional expression create inadequate interpersonal communication. Laurenceau et al. (1998), found that self-disclosure, other disclosure, and disclosure responsiveness at an interaction-by-interaction level were the most significant components to the formation of intimacy between people. It can become difficult to love a person when that person is difficult to get to know in a deeper more intimate way through disclosure and responsiveness (Derlega, 2013; Mashek & Aron, 2004). All NT interviewees within the study revealed they felt that the needs of their ASC partner/family members were being met to some extent; however, their needs remained fully unmet. The lack of expected warmth and intimacy within their relationships not only had a detrimental effect on their ability to grow close to their partner/family members, but a needs deprivation meant that the relationship lacked the warmth and depth that they needed:

> NORA   *I think … I always sensed that I had a soul and a deep sense of self at some level and I always thought that in my mind that I would experience really deep enriching relationships that would get deeper with time and that there'd be a certain emotional intimacy that*

> *would grow in relationships and that growth emotional intimacy will just never happen with my husband.*

HOLLY   *So all of those things have kind of damaged any intimacy we would have because … right through our relationship has been a lack of trust because his words were not consistent with his behaviour.*

WANDA   *The to and fro of ideas and listening to others, whereas with my relationship with Wally it's sometimes hard to have an ongoing conversation because it seems that there always has to be a right or wrong answer … one thing that you might say is going to lead to something else, but he jumps on the first thing that you've said and … takes that very literally, you might have been sort of trying to express yourself in a more long-winded way which I usually do ha, ha …*

Basically, Wally (ASC) agreed with Wanda:

I'm probably not very good at recognising what or how to offer emotional support. I've learnt to back off a little bit and just to listen, but unfortunately that sometimes becomes unresponsive in that she'll say that 'I'm telling you all this stuff and I'm getting nothing back' and I'm like 'Well I don't know what to give you because I don't have any answers' is what I've said in the past … I don't have any answers to that and all I can do is listen.

Have They Gone Nuts?

Participants with ASC, discussed the challenges of being required to offer emotional support, share in meaningful conversation, and cultivate intimacy in their relationships. Mary described how she used a script to work out how to react in any given situation:

> *I work with a script. And this big fast brain of mine is a massive database. I have taken all instructions and knowledge from whatever. I've watched people, interacted with people, watched TV shows, read books. Anything that I think I can apply, I will absorb and I put in this database, and then when I come up against something, I will apply a script to it, and I will think – okay in this instance, or when this happened before to that person in that TV show, book, past life experience, whatever, this is what they did, and I will apply it. And life doesn't really work that way all the time, so it's just like that saying, I think it was Einstein, that doing the same thing and expecting a different outcome. It's a form of madness or insanity. So oftentimes I will go and apply the same thing over and over again to the same issue and expecting a different outcome, because – like it worked before so the probability of it working again is quite high. Why isn't this happening? Because I don't take in the variable which is the human being and human beings are funny.*

Other ASC participants shared how making improvements in conversational intimacy meant unwelcome effort on their part:

> *RICHARD*   *It's been a frustrating exercise ... I'll give one, or two, word answers, whereas she's looking for ... talk[ing] it out a bit more, but as I say that's more ... effort on my part.*

A Collision of Needs

RACHELLE *I don't think he is happy at all ... I don't answer the way he wants me to answer from an emotional point of view ... I don't really know how to ... sometimes I need like a third party like my mum or Ryan's mum or someone to explain it to me what it all means and ... if we're dealing with a big issue we tend to have the same conversation a few times before I understand what he wants.*

Alternatively, Rachelle's husband Ryan (NT) said:

Conversations when they get down to deep and meaningful things often bog down in a kind of a situation where she has expressed needs, and wants to focus on those being met and often what I want are uncounted ... a deep and meaningful conversation is often a fourth conversation ... so that you sort of bite the bullet and just live with that and some of that it, over time ... resolves itself anyway.

Some ASC participants struggled with attempts to solve the conversational intimacy divide:

TOM *[He] has drawn me into deep conversations about feelings when he needed to resolve something. While the conversations were difficult for me, the result was good. I can recall times when I made an emotional response to something that angered me. This resulted in extended periods of discomfort. I see the value in trying to have a non-angry conversation about things that bother me. However, this type of conversation is still difficult for me, and I don't like it.*

81

TERRY   *I don't telegraph the right signals because I don't reflect what she wants to see in me because I don't read her emotional state very well at all.*

EDITH   *Never guaranteed to be able to do it, I never know that I can do that and I don't necessarily know how my efforts will be received because … I can't read the body language well enough to know, but I sort of want to keep on going and when something gets difficult and I feel wronged or I feel not understood I'll keep on pushing and I know I shouldn't.*

DANIEL   *I make stilted comments that sometimes get across. I share looks, touch, hugs, sometimes.*

In Summary

Stemming from the main differences that autistic people have in the areas of social interaction, social reciprocity and social imagination (American Psychiatric Association, 2013), neurodiverse relationships experience a distinct shortage of personal interaction, especially the emotional, affectionate, deep and meaningful modes of conversation. This feature shaped a distinctive type of relationship; one in which there were much lower levels of warmth and affection than usual. Consequently, the people involved experienced diametrically opposed needs.

A Collision of Needs

Participants with ASC disclosed how their need to disengage from interaction set in motion a desire for company but without any emotional conversation. This objective was achieved by withdrawing from all conversations that required personal or deep and meaningful conversation. Withdrawing to a place of solitude to relieve tensions or by taking refuge in spending time with special interests were chosen by most ASC participants. However, these actions were found to be unacceptable by most NT participants. Their need for their relationships to include reciprocated expressive and deep conversations that led to a deep connectedness with pleasant amounts of conversational intimacy were mostly left wanting. Instead, superficial conversations became the custom, which was insufficient for their needs.

In the next chapter, participants shared how these extensive needs incompatibilities undermined abilities for each to grow together. An ever-widening gulf opened between them. Often these incompatibilities became a primary source of conflict.

5

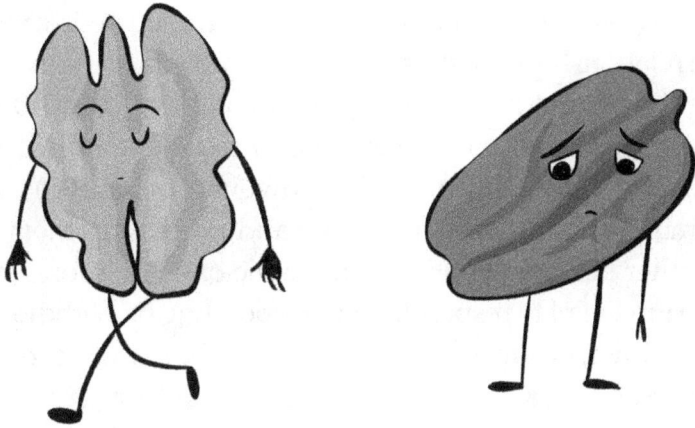

Facing
A Different Page

Have They Gone Nuts?

'If we have no peace, it is because we have forgotten that we belong to each other.'
Mother Teresa

On Different Pages

There is clear evidence that the most satisfied people within close relationships are those who do not avoid communication about important relational topics or conflicts – instead they develop a sense of working together through their difficulties (Gottman & Gottman, 2017). However, difficulties with communication, social interaction and processing their own and other people's emotions can be the basis for those on the spectrum to fail to respond, avoid responding by withdrawing and, at times, desire a withdrawal from all communication for extended periods of time (Attwood, 2015; Gillberg et al., 2015). Although trying to find a resolution when conflict occurred was the aim of most NT participants, working through difficulties together was not the aim of ASC participants. The pairing of incompatible needs and incompatible ways to meet those needs between the two groups of people was found to be the catalyst that often led to unresolvable differences. The communication difficulties, the shortage of passionate and explicit expressions of love and care, the desires for different styles of conversation, and different requirements for solitude often created a problem-solving divide. Wally could not see the point in resolving disagreements with his partner:

Maybe it was unresolved, but we can't keep hammering away at something until it's resolved because some of these things are unresolvable.

Facing A Different Page

Many ASC participants described that their lack of conversational success drove them to escape difficult conversations rather than endeavour to resolve them. Stella explained why this was the case for her:

> *I also become completely lost when conversation becomes very emotional and can hardly listen. I become so overwhelmed ... that I understand nothing and have no idea what to say.*

Ronald decided it was better to communicate without words:

> *I would communicate by taking some sort of action rather than talk about it.*

Some ASC participants mentioned that their multiple failures did not help their self-esteem. Phil referred to this aspect:

> *Ah, it doesn't do anything for the confidence ... or the ability to do things ... It just puts your confidence down, in your abilities.*

However, he shared that he was trying hard to find ways to work towards a better way of interacting:

> *Yeah ... I keep trying to ask questions until I can understand what it is that went wrong. Half the time I just don't know ... Sometimes I have to ask questions and try and figure out what went wrong so that I can apologise or whatever ... do something.*

On the other hand, NT participants look to solve problems so that they can move on. While Dawn's dissatisfaction was evident, her words revealed that it was her partner's lack of awareness of both his behaviour, and how his behaviour affected her that were most upsetting:

> *If we are in a conversation and I said 'I am very unhappy because ... ' or 'your behaviour was ... ' he will react saying 'well you did such and such' ... He never says, 'I am unhappy with you because ... ' or 'I am uncomfortable ... ' or 'can we talk about this ... '. Never, NEVER.*

Similarly, Ruth shared her frustrations:

> *It seems like every time I THINK we are on the same page, I come to find out that we are not ... We will discuss an important matter ... he will agree with me ... on a course of action, and then a few days later he won't follow the plan we had discussed. When he does this, I don't really feel like following it either because I say to myself 'What is the point when he just goes off and does B again instead of what we talked about and agreed to?' It looks rather selfish to me when he does this. His reasons make sense to him, but not to me. I feel unheard and disrespected, and then we do it all over again with the next important conversation.*

Rose agreed with this sentiment:

> *In conversations I guess the biggest challenge is ... if we're taking it in two different directions and especially if I get frustrated about it because Pierre is already trying really hard ... I feel bad because I know it's not really fair to him and it's just a miscommunication but I get really frustrated because I do really want to be going from the same page.*

Wanda described the many complexities to attempting to deal with problems:

I do try ... and that is a relationship problem ... what you're trying to bring up by saying how you're feeling and they basically seem to just ignore it and carry on that 'Yeah oh you obviously were just having a bad day or something.' ... It doesn't solve the problem ... every time something happens where you've had a major falling out about something it's like another little piece of you kind of dissolves or disintegrates or shuts off or something.

Comments from a survey respondent with ASC demonstrated that to be on the same page with others held little merit:

Now I have had so much therapy and social skills training, that I now go through the motions to get on with people, and wear an invisible mask each day, and do things that aren't authentic, to keep everyone else happy and get ahead in life. Do I believe what I am doing – no. I don't believe it. It is important to other people, so I am faking it. It is important to other people to take turns, so I do it. I don't believe it as something important to me, rather it is something important to other people that I fake because I want something out of that other person – information, speed in processing my request, etc.

In contrast, a comment from a male NT survey respondent shared that he had a longing to succeed in the endeavour of sustaining the quality of his relationship, however, he struggled with the one-sidedness of this responsibility; a viewpoint shared by many NT participants in the study:

I am at a loss as to how to improve the relationship. Neither talking it out, or not talking about it, seem to work. It's like, rather than having two individual agendas and one agreed upon cumulative agenda, there is her agenda and – at best – my agenda items are footnotes at the bottom of the page in superscript.

Loving Blind

The term 'Theory of Mind' describes the processes in the brain that are involved in understanding that other people have independent mental states, such as beliefs, desires, intentions, imagination and emotions, and this understanding is then used to identify and predict the behaviour of others. Baron-Cohen (2008) describes Theory of Mind (ToM) as 'the ability to put oneself into someone else's shoes, to imagine their thoughts and feelings' (p. 112). A limited ToM (often referred to as mind-blindness) is one of the characteristic features of the ASCs (Baron-Cohen, 1997). For individuals to connect, communicate and fully take part in the social world it is important to have an intact ToM. It provides that social 'know-how', that instinctive 'knowing' of how to react in any given situation. The interviews revealed that many ASC participants showed a noticeable lack of awareness about their limitations with interaction. This lack of awareness prevented many from taking responsibility for communication difficulties, or figuring out a different way of interacting in their relationships. Sharon (ASC) said that other people were the cause of the communication issues she experienced with others:

I guess, in general, people don't like it when other people point out that they are the cause of an ineffective communication.

Similarly, Cora (ASC) felt unfairly blamed:

> *Yes. But he seemed to believe it was only me who had to seek help, as he pinned the blame of all our difficulties on me and my ASD.*

However, Derek (NT) (Cora's partner) conveyed a different view:

> *She never knew that she had Asperger's until we were together ... I was ... wondering why it is that we just can't seem to have ... a proper conventional, rational conversation. It seems that we had a conversation and then we both walk away, and then she sees it completely different to what we, what I thought that we just agreed to ... this sort of elementary miscommunication that is going on ... it's not that she's thick, because I have seen her be quite smart ... and she said to me a couple of times, 'I don't think I think like other people' and I just sort of took that on board and started having a look around ... some of the possibilities then came from autism, ... Asperger's ... and at the same time Cora was also looking up, following up leads from an ... aunt that had a similar sort of behavioural difficulty and so ... then we sort of found out.*

Jim (ASC) felt that the difficulties between Dianne (NT) and him were due to her work, or her lack of sleep, rather than the communication problems between them:

> *She ... gets frustrated at work with the people that she works for and ... she brings it home ... so I cop it all the time ... I just shut up and walk away, and of course that stirs her even more ... because Dianne wants ... a good working*

relationship in regards to communication ... she has often ... said 'I don't understand you' ... she says that I make this as an excuse, but I don't think she gets enough sleep.

On the other hand, Dianne (NT) recognised that it was the communication problems between them that caused their difficulties:

I just tell him he sucks actually. I have done that before ... I have always told him that he has never had to guess about how I feel. I have always told him ... 'Look, this is what I need from you.' And I can think back, way before he was even diagnosed, in our relationship, having those conversations with him, you know. 'I need more of you.' 'You don't give me enough of yourself.' 'You don't talk to me about you.' And being very honest ... I say this is not fair, this is not. I explained that I don't think this is what a relationship should be ... Those things need to happen, and because they don't, this is why we don't have this relationship.

Holly (NT) summed up the issue:

It usually most obviously comes out in the send and receive. What I think I've sent and what I think I've received often show up to be afterwards, not.

A Predicament of Perceptions

The two groups of participants showed a distinct awareness gulf about the respective feelings of satisfaction or dissatisfaction. Although NT participants reported that their satisfaction of affection and connection was quite low and that they did not withhold this fact from their ASC partner/family members, ASC participants showed very limited understanding of these views. A common conclusion for NT participants was to question whether their partner/family member felt any affection for them. However, these doubts caused some concerns for a few ASC participants. Murray (ASC) noted:

> *My wife points out that my ... levels of affection aren't what she would expect normally ... it's very easy for someone to assume that that means that they don't love you as much because you're not as affectionate as they would expect.*

Most NT participants discussed at length their belief that the low levels of affection and connection would not be considered typical by the general population. It was especially so, when they experienced resistance to their efforts to make changes and increase affection and connection. Although NT participants realised that many of the reasons for the resistance was due to the difficulties and differences of autism, and so it was often unintentional, they expressed dismay at their partner/family member's reluctance to amend the situation, even moderately for them. It appeared to them that their partner/family member with ASC were reasonably contented with the lower amounts of affection and connection. Participants with ASC confirmed that were content to leave things as they were:

> SHARON *In my previous marriage to NT-partner, I have found that our expectations and requirements for emotional connection were quite different. I was craving more personal space and time, while he was wanting to do many things together.*

TOM   *I feel comfortable when I am with Ken and I do not feel lonely. To me that is a satisfactory emotional connection. I don't know how to make warm affectionate conversations, but I don't feel anything lacking. Sometimes Ken says our intimacy is lacking.*

An anonymous comment from an ASC survey respondent suggests a lack of awareness that a 'decline' in his relationship might have something to do his particular difficulties:

I am a man with Asperger's (high functioning). I have serious suspicions that my partner is on the spectrum. She refuses to be diagnosed. I sometimes feel as though I am the normal one, cause I know that Aspies should have issues with stuff that I often don't, but some of the issues that we are having are because she is emotionally unavailable, not me. As a result of this and other factors this is what I would consider a declining relationship with no prospect of continuing romantically, however we do want to remain friends just in a more distant capacity.

Unable to change their partner/family members perceptions, as time went on, NT participants became more and more dissatisfied:

NORA   *When I say to him 'Are you happy?' He goes 'Yeah, I've got no problems with you. This is great for me, this relationship.' I'm like 'I'm glad you're so happy.'*

SABRINA   *The affection stayed for a little while, but then, it just gradually fell off … and he doesn't seem*

>to be that bothered by it, so that's kind of the
>sad part.

RENEE   *I think he's reasonably happy about it because he*
        doesn't need that level of emotional connection
        really, or he doesn't appear to ... the fact is I'm
        his wife, we've been married for coming up 33
        years, as long as things are okay in his world,
        then he thinks that it's okay in my world.

LAURA   *The warmth and affection is a one-way street;*
        I should give it to him and be content that he
        solicits/accepts it ... He does not seem to want
        or solicit greater connection.

DIANNE *If the relationship was one where it was a*
        caring, sharing relationship but ... I feel like
        I'm living, boarding in a house with somebody
        who is not paying their half of the rent.

However, Mia's comments illustrated variations do exist within neurodiverse relationships. She described how her relationship was distinctively unique to most neurodiverse relationships in the study and, so, she appeared to be more satisfied in her relationship than most NT participants in the study:

I'm satisfied in our relationship, particularly in regards to
understanding the ways that Max expresses love in that he
likes to connect, he likes conversation, he likes to talk about
current events and world events and he is a good listener
and, yeah, so I think we do share a good connection in that
we talk, we spend time together, it's give and take.

Have They Gone Nuts?

Confirming Mia's comments, her husband, Max (ASC) gave his viewpoint on reasons why their satisfaction levels appeared to surpass the average neurodiverse relationship. Also, regarding Murray's earlier comments about his wife's doubts because *'his levels of affection aren't what she would expect normally'*, Max's description gave a possible explanation as to why many NT adults experience doubts about their partner/ family members' affection:

> *I've had a lot of training with Mia. She's really helped me know what ... to do and ... our relationship has improved tremendously ... My natural response is to be Mr Blank Face, Mr Poker Face, and to not interact, not even smile and interestingly ... when I focus on what someone is saying I will lose all expression in the face ... and ... create the impression in the other person's mind that I'm not paying attention to them, when in fact I'm extra paying attention to them ... One of the things Mia did was ... 'don't do ear only listening' because that's what I do, ear only, and lose other aspects of visual feedback to show that I'm actually paying attention ... but I guess if you don't have that desire to learn or ... willingness to learn, then that itself would be an impediment to learning.*

In Summary

It is well known that the social interaction needs of those with ASC differ significantly from the NT population (Mendes, 2015). In these studies, these different needs were found to create an incompatible relational dynamic. The needs of one to have an abundance of emotional interaction and build warmth and connection was diametrically opposed to the needs of the other to have a great deal of solitude and silence. The result of this pairing of incompatible needs within a relationship was a power struggle as each tried to get their opposing need met, which in turn, triggered a multitude of unresolvable differences.

Participants with ASC coped by becoming unresponsive to their partner/family members. While many ASC participants openly discussed their unresponsive, withdrawal and avoidant behaviours, they appeared to be unaware that these behaviours not only prevented their partner/family members' efforts to connect with, and collaborate with them, but also resulted in their own relationship dissatisfaction. When considering mind-blindness (Baron-Cohen, 1997), with the associated lack of awareness, connecting their dissatisfaction with their own behaviour may be challenging for those with ASC. Connecting their dissatisfaction with their partner/ family members' behaviour however, has the potential to proliferate impressions of being misunderstood, uncared for and mistrusted to each other, and by each other. Some ASC participants accepted that they were not good at giving emotional support, or recognising the necessity, but they did not appear to consider that an increase in their efforts would improve unresolvable differences.

On the other hand, NT participants reported that the low intensities of affection created challenges that were difficult to surmount for them, especially when experiencing resistance to their efforts to make changes. However, while ASC participants were satisfied with lower levels of affection, NT participants were not. The effect of this satisfaction difference of opinion was inequitable intentions towards change. The NT group wanted an improvement to affection and connection intensities, whereas the ASC group were content to leave things as they were. Some ASC participants indicated that they would be content with even lower quantities of affection and connection than currently existed in their relationship.

The differences between each group triggered contrasting compensatory strategies. Adults with ASC tried to counteract their communication difficulties through avoidance of conversation, evading interpersonal questions and limiting responses. However, many misinterpretations and assumptions resulted. In contrast, NT adults tried to counteract the avoidance tactics of their partner/ family members with prompting, guiding and directing conversations, together with extensive conversation preparation. The strength and amount of conversation preparations that were required were very atypical for close relationships. These contrasting compensatory strategies are discussed in the next chapter.

6

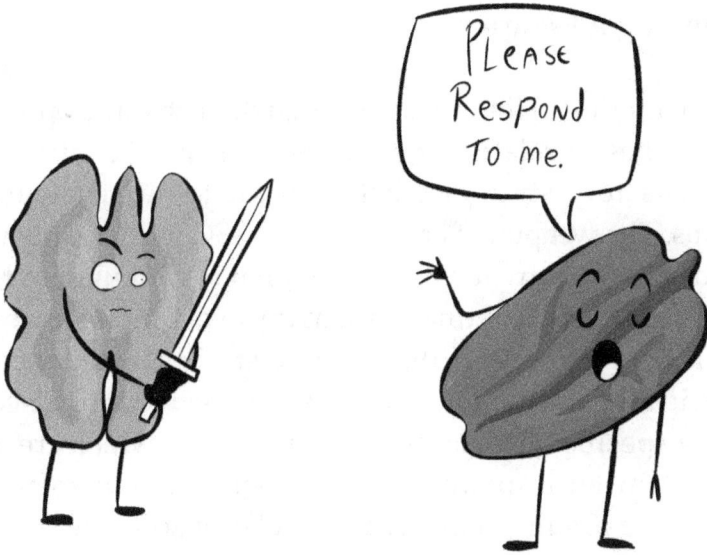

Slaying the
Dragon of Difference

'It is not our differences that divide us.
It is our inability to recognise, accept and
celebrate those differences.'
Audre Lorde

Choosing a Weapon

Attempting to find a way through diametrically opposed approaches to relating was found to trigger contrasting compensatory strategies between the two participating groups. The weapon of choice for the ASC participants was avoidance in many forms. Although it is well known that people with ASC routinely use many avoidant behaviours (Egan & Linenberg, 2019), in these studies, avoidance of participating in emotional conversations led to avoidance of asking specific types of personal questions, which created a problem with misinterpreting actions, and forming inaccurate assumptions in their relationships. Since the thinking of those on the autism spectrum are generally 'reality-based rather than imaginative' (Craig & Baron-Cohen, 1999, p. 325), this type of thinking affects abilities to be aware of others' thoughts, feelings and reasonings, and increases the likelihood of misunderstanding the intent of others. Consequently, the similar outcomes of both conversation avoidance and reality-based thinking fortify each other. When including unresponsiveness, the combination of these behaviours not only prevents the efforts of others to connect with, and collaborate with them, but also can result in their own relationship dissatisfaction (Egan & Linenberg, 2019; Gottman, 1993). However, in these studies, the dissatisfaction that participants with

ASC experienced in their relationships were mainly due to the propensity their NT partner/family members had to challenge their avoidance behaviours. Therefore, while avoidance and unresponsiveness were used to get out of unwanted situations, the desired effect rarely occurred.

On the other hand, NT participants chose prompting, as their weapon of choice. The intent was to gain affectionate conversation and connection or resolve issues that arose from their ASC partner/family member's unresponsive and avoidance strategies. Attempts to counter the self-protective behaviours employed by their partner/family members often involved extra communicational effort for NT participants through prompting, guiding and directing conversations.

A Sword of Self-Protection

A lack of involvement in the crucial features of interpersonal conversations, such as displaying verbal interest in another's conversation by questioning and probing the speaker's meanings and giving comfort and support through asking questions were common behaviours shown by participants with ASC. When accompanied by the many avoidance behaviours participants with ASC used, the result was a distinct absence of asking interpersonal questions; misinterpreting actions; and forming inaccurate assumptions. While the intended outcome of these avoidance behaviours was to cope with conversation inabilities, and consequently, avoid emotional conversation, it appeared that an often-unintended outcome was that these self-protective strategies became triggers for the compensatory strategies that the NT participants used.

Question and Response Avoidance

Accounts provided by ASC participants illustrate that stonewalling behaviour (i.e. avoiding conversations, becoming defensive, shutting down and becoming verbally aggressive) offered protection for them. Rather than ask questions, these behaviours supplied the opportunity to withdraw from difficult and unwanted conversations. Despite this, reports given by both groups of participants showed that this avoidance often increased the interaction that they were trying to avoid since NT participants wanted to find answers to their questions and encourage the emotional connection they were looking for. Richard confirmed that while he could see something was 'wrong' he preferred to turn a blind eye, not ask questions, and, therefore, protect himself. His answer also revealed that he lacked the awareness that his avoidance of answering his partner's questions increased the likelihood that 'her pushing' and asking would continue:

> *But if I can sort of see something is wrong, I don't ask questions ... She requires an answer ... pushing and pushing ... It gets too annoying, sometimes an argument.*

Terry showed insight that asking questions and asking for clarification would help him understand better; still he revealed that he did not often recognise when to ask for clarification:

> *Kim would like me to take the lead with conversation at times and ask questions rather than hang back ... If she says something that I take literally ... [or] I don't understand and I need more information ... to actually stop and ask for clarification.*

Slaying the Dragon of Difference

The interconnected life that NT participants longed to share with their partner/family members was a frequent casualty of the lack of interpersonal questions. However, their need to be emotionally connected with their partner/family members meant that starting interaction and asking questions themselves was unavoidable:

RUTH
Most of our conversations are exchanges of information. He has learned to ask me questions like 'How are you doing', 'How was your day' ... but again, those things have not come naturally to him ... He doesn't usually go there to the 'why' behind things himself. I usually have to ask him questions. He needs instructions, so if I provide them, he can usually follow them in his own way ... I feel like I am the one who mostly starts conversations unless he has some information for me. Even when he does have important things he needs to tell me, I have to 'figure it out' and sit and ask him question after question after question until I get an answer. I feel like I have to read him or read his mind pretty often because he's not going to volunteer information.

DAWN
If there is something that needs to be talked about, I'm the one that brings it up ... it doesn't cross his mind to talk to me about stuff, whether it is what he is doing at work, or what we are supposed to be doing next month.

RONDA
A major piece of the relationship that was sorely missing was that someone who

> *would spontaneously come and seek me,*
> *seek my presence, seek my opinion, seek my*
> *companionship, you know invite me, 'let's go*
> *to a movie' or 'let's do something', or 'how*
> *are you doing', you know 'what's going on?'*
> *No. Zero seeking on his part.*

Mandy gave an example of how confusing a conversation can become due to her husband's lack of question asking and answering abilities:

> *He won't come to me and say 'You're cranky. What's wrong?'*
> *He will just go about his day and that would just go on for*
> *days and days. There would be no chatting about anything.*
> *So, if I want to make it work, I have to either go to him, or*
> *find a solution, or learn to tuck my stuff away, because it's*
> *not going to solve anything. It's not going to fix anything*
> *… Even just organisational skills. I'm always in trouble for*
> *asking too many questions but if I don't ask, I don't know*
> *anything. If something has moved, then I have to ask where*
> *it's gone. It's like 'Well it's away' and it's like 'Yeah but*
> *where did you put it?' 'Why do you have to know? I've put*
> *it away.' But most of the time it's not where it should be and*
> *I, then, can't find it the next time I need it, so it's like you're*
> *constantly managing … Sometimes it's a bit like a puzzle.*
> *So, you don't get all the pieces of what they're saying. So,*
> *you've got to try and put it together and sometimes they miss,*
> *it's like Chinese instructions, they miss a line in between.*
> *So, you're trying to work out how to put the conversation*
> *together and how it has relevance to what you're talking*
> *about … It's hard to explain unless you use examples, but*
> *if you say to him:*

'Did you use the scissors?' and he'll say 'Yes.'
So ... 'Where did you leave them?'
'Well, I didn't have them last.'
'So, where did you put them when you used them?'
'Well, they go in the drawer.'
'Okay, well they're not in the drawer. Where did you actually do the present?'
'Why?'
'Because I want to have a look.'
'Well, I didn't have them last. How do you know someone else hasn't used them?'

So, you're still just trying to find out where they were or what they were doing at the time so that you can go back and retrace the steps and then maybe find what you're looking for.

Misinterpretations and Assumptions

Inaccurate assumptions were found to be based on ASC participants' predisposition towards misinterpreting what others said and did. A tendency to avoid the types of conversations that would normally support working together on relationship problems and sustain a relationship, increased the likelihood of getting things wrong. While this avoidance was used for self-protective means, a frequent result was a decreasing commitment to the relationship. This combination of conversation avoidance, misinterpretations and inaccurate assumptions become part of an overall conversation avoidance pattern which, for participants with ASC, seemed to become their dominant compensatory strategy in avoidance of the affectionate and/or personal conversations that their NT partner/family members were looking for. Inaccurate assumptions were also found to influence a considerable number of interactions in their relationships. Participants with ASC illustrated that they were either unaware that they had formed an assumption or did not know how to put right misunderstandings after forming an assumption. They also seemed unaware that investing time into becoming more effective within conversations by asking questions and proactively listening could correct inaccurate assumptions. Barry shared that he analysed what was being said, rather than listening to what was said:

> *I suppose there's times … for instance she says something, I'm inclined to listen to the first part and then go off on a tangent, analysing that and then not hearing what she is saying after that, and she might take that as meaning that I am not interested but, but I am, or I am trying to do two things at once. Like … I'm in the midst of something and she is talking and I'm thinking 'Well I can't do both of these' so I will pretend I am hearing and I will say yes, yes, yes to anything and then she will realise it, because I can't be saying yes to everything.*

Rachelle assumed that others talk to hear themselves:

> *I just try and withdraw from conversation at work because people tend to talk about the same things over and over again … it's so shallow and minor as well. They're just talking to hear their own voices sometimes.*

Many NT participants reported that they felt a lack of questions and not listening to them were the main reasons for the substantial inaccurate assumptions that occurred in their relationships and that, as a result, conversations, actions and events were repeatedly misconstrued. Rather than being able to communicate their commitment to each other and grow their relationship, misunderstanding and difficulties occurred on a regular basis. Dawn shared her experiences of her partner's propensity to form assumptions based on his misinterpretation of events, and the effect it had on her life:

He takes away what can be a completely different perception of what I have said ... he doesn't ask me anything, my feelings or thoughts on things and then makes sweeping assumptions, I mean I have heard him telling somebody, 'Oh Dawn thinks blah, blah, blah' and I am like 'I never said that. Where did that come from?' ... That's not uncommon, and he has ... obviously heard my voice in his head saying 'Dawn likes A' instead of asking Dawn if she likes A or B and finding out that she likes B and so he makes these sweeping assumptions ... without checking on them first.

Like Dawn, Maggie described her husband having conversations with her in his head. She revealed the strategies that she implemented to cope with the aftermaths of incorrect assumptions, both from her daughter and her husband:

My husband has conversations with me in his head and then vows and declares that that's what I've said and I used to think I was going crazy because I don't remember these conversations until I worked it out ... but for Chloe I have to have things written down which is why I like the text ... if she says one thing and then she says another I can turn round and say 'No you said this, see, check the text message that you said it,' and she'll check it and go 'Oh!' ... I've noticed with Luke, he will grab on to part of what I've said and run with that and think he knows what I'm talking about.

Have They Gone Nuts?

Ronda made an interesting point about how misinterpretations can occur:

> *Some researchers ... said [that] a major source of their social misunderstandings is because they jump to conclusions too quickly and they jump to the wrong conclusion.*

Holly commented on her husband's tendency to assume he understood which led to her assume that he understood as well:

> *Jack's very compliant. He wants to please you, so he will be very agreeable and that masked the fact that he actually didn't understand, or couldn't compute what was actually required of him ... If he did a task, let's say planting a plant for me, he might dig the hole and we'd have a discussion about how it should be done and I would leave him to do it and I would come back and he would have done it in a different way and then that would provoke a fight and when I would say 'Well I said dah, dah, dah, dah, dah' and he'd say, 'Oh yes, but I thought you meant dah, dah, dah, dah, dah.' Then this digression would occur, and the problem was I never knew that he hadn't taken the meaning I had given after all the time he's in front of me going yeah, yeah, yeah, yep, and not until the physical evidence was there would I know, so I guess that's probably happened in our relationship too, of where I might have thought he took a meaning from something I said or did and he hadn't.*

Georgia complained about the results of her husband's assumptions:

I ended up handling all the bills and he said, 'Well I just assumed you wanted control.' And I was like 'Shit NO! I would have loved you to have helped me with this. It's really stressful!!' But he assumed because I was doing it, that I wanted to do it ... and I then look at myself and say well I could've asked ... but then something happened in me where I just became reticent and I'm wondering if its built on history where you are constantly having to ask, you're having to ask for things to be done, you're having to ask for a reaction, you're having to ask for participation in the family, you're having to initiate everything so you get to a point where you just stop asking and you allow them to run with their assumptions because it's just easier.

A Sword of Prompting

Affectionate communication is a key characteristic of healthy close relationships – and one of the usual signs of a failing relationship is a lack of it. According to Hesse (2020) affection deprivation, which occurs when people desire more affection than they are currently receiving, has significant influence on mental and relational wellbeing. Hesse's (2020) study of marital relationships found that the amount of affection given 'matters far beyond the relationship itself' (p. 980). Affectionate communication, therefore, not only has important connotations for relationship health, but also the health and wellbeing of the individuals concerned.

Prompting

Prompting was the main approach used by NT participants intended to trigger responses and activate reciprocal affectionate interaction. Prompts took the form of reminders, instructions and explanations, and were expected to resolve the lack of responsiveness they experienced from their partners and family members with ASC and improve affectionate and personal interaction. The belief was that the necessity to prompt would cease. However, it was found that this strategy, while only partially successful in the attainment of the intended outcomes, continued to be a requirement, rather than coming to an end. NT participants reported that the desired outcomes were often thwarted by a chain of behaviours exhibited by their partners/family members with ASC that prevented communication. These behaviours also negated further interaction. When not able to avoid unwanted interaction, ASC adults became dependent on the prompts that helped their responses. Unprompted responding only occasionally improved. Hazel (NT) noted the very specific communication differences that occurs in neurodiverse relationships as opposed to typical relationships:

> *I know that in a NT/NT relationship, they get each other and even though there are differences with man and the wife, they actually understand each other and don't have to go the long route of explaining actions or explaining why they want to do something ... Whereas with us, there is a lot of explanation needed and when communication is not good, which in this case, it is not good, always, then you just have to guess why they are doing that particular thing that way. Whereas in a neurotypical/neurotypical relationship, they would understand right away why they are doing something*

*that way and if they didn't understand the other person,
they could communicate by saying 'Why did you do that?'*

Terry (ASC) commented on the ways in which his partner
prompted him and instructed him in the customs of reciprocal
interaction:

*If she does notice that I'm doing or stretching myself to try
something once I take a pause to think about what I'm going
to do or say next she may interject with 'Well now you're
supposed to ask me about this or perhaps you should consider
that.' So, if she's in the mood she will prompt me for more.*

Participants with ASC revealed that they understood
that their partner/family members wanted more meaningful
conversation and, therefore, often prompted conversations
to occur and/or continue with them. Regardless of this
realisation, they openly acknowledged that they often chose
not to take part in these conversations. Participants with ASC
often saw the situation as an issue of their partner/family
members, rather than because of something that they needed
to address. Consequently, many ASC participants appeared
to find their partner/family members attempts to initiate
conversation and connection unnecessary, or a hindrance.
Samuel's words implied as much:

*I would find the prompting about that sort of thing would be
annoying … I don't find it necessary to continue on because
her conversations go into what I consider unnecessary detail
and repetitiveness.*

Then he added other instances of his 'annoyance' at his
partner's prompts:

In a lot of cases I would take our previous discussion as an agreement whereas she would take it as a discussion and … we still hadn't actually come to a conclusion, according to her. I would find the prompting about that sort of thing would be annoying in a sense in the fact that I thought we'd agreed on something and she's saying no we hadn't.

Murray admitted that his emotional responsiveness only occurred when his partner elicits it from him:

To be honest it's probably usually reactive, so she'll display affection towards me, so I'll try to display affection back. I'm not usually proactive in displaying affection.

Although Stella indicated that she noticed her partner's attempts to bring about more emotional conversations between them, she did not respond. Instead, she assumed that his displeasure, and not her lack of response, was the reason for his prompts:

I sometimes notice his efforts, but they annoy me, as I either want to be left alone or I need a different way of connection … Yes, he has prompted conversations, usually straight away, when he was displeased with my behaviour/words.

Daniel described how his partner had 'trained' him to respond, however, he expressed a tendency to do the opposite:

Cathy takes care to get my attention and tells me what she has to say clearly. I'm trained to wait for her to solicit a response, although I am prone to interrupt. I'm trained too, to answer the question she's asked. Humiliating but effective … Letting go of frustration helps … My natural tendency is to fall silent.

Slaying the Dragon of Difference

Most NT participants reported that an inability to obtain the emotional connection they needed was a major difficulty for them. However, most revealed a desire to persist in their endeavours to overcome the difficulties. This desire escalated as awareness of the ASC condition increased. Since their partner/family members did not initiate emotional connection, but prompting did achieve some successful interaction, at times, prompting became the main approach used to achieve their goal. All NT interviewees discussed many different prompting strategies that they used, with the main course of action being to use questions, instructions, directions or explanations. For example, Ruth found that connection with her partner was possible if she kept prompting with questions:

> With prompting, my husband tries to put forth the effort to connect with me, not just share information. I am the one who has to ask him questions in an effort to connect. He doesn't go out of his way to connect with me.

Then she added:

> I wish I didn't have to prompt him ... but I realise that is the reality of my life ... He needs instructions, so if I provide them, he can usually follow them in his own way ... It would be great if he could say these things without prompting, but I know that may never happen.

Dianne reported that, rather than talk about it, she used a range of non-verbal methods to prompt such as lists:

> If things need to be done, I write a list of tasks to be done 'cause, they are not good planners, and if I don't put a list

*down to go, 'These things need to be done', he would just
sort of kind of fart around for the day.*

Shirley described the frustration she felt by being required to
find the 'right' questions to get the answers that she wanted:

*In order for me to get the information I want I have to be
very specific about how I prompt her with my questions to
give me the information, if I don't ask the right questions
then I won't get that information voluntarily. So, she's not
going to sit on the couch and say 'Oh I had a really hard
client today that came in and this is what happened' … If I
said to her when she got home 'How was your day? Did you
have any rough clients, or did you have any hard clients?'
Then the story will come out. So, sometimes with Jill it's
like getting blood from a stone … If I don't ask the right
question, I won't get the information spontaneously which
is sometimes extremely frustrating that I have to try and
guess what the questions are, but yeah, she finds it really
hard to enter spontaneous conversations about her day so
yes, I do have to prompt a lot.*

Kay gave examples of her course of action that involved
prompting through a pattern of positive reminders:

*'Did you understand what I was feeling or what I meant
before? Or how that went?' so it is constantly going back
and reminding and reminding this is what happened. This
is how I felt. This is what I need. Again. And can we move
forward and have an agreed way forward? And consistently
going back to that. Going back to that until it is almost like
a habit.*

Alex explained that prompting increased the likelihood that Mary would take part in the social activities that she avoided:

Well, the communication I guess, it is not me trying to talk her into it but maybe trying to outline the benefits of maybe doing it, whether it be a social thing with friends, or just going to someone's house for dinner where she doesn't want to. And usually … she walks away and she is knackered but she goes 'Oh wow, I had a really good time' … And that is sort of what I guess I am trying to communicate with her is like 'Do you remember the last time where, as much as you hate the thought of it before we are there, but once you are there you seem to sort of, click and enjoy yourself?' … So that's about it. It is more trying to outline the benefits of doing something like that. What she will get out of it.

Dawn said that that she felt like a 'nag' due to the requirement to prompt:

I've learnt not to expect normal communication about information. I have to ask, and I have learnt to accept that I may sound like a nosy nag but if I don't ask I won't get told.

When participants with ASC were asked if they had felt a need to prompt conversations for connection to occur, most answered no. However, a few described reasons that they may occasionally use prompting within their conversations:

SAMUEL   *Yeah, few and far between. I don't generally prompt conversation apart from the necessary small talk to get on together.*

TERRY   *The only time I've needed to prompt her is if*
         she is in a bad mood and I'm trying to make
         up because it's quite likely she's in a bad mood
         because of something I've done or said, or not
         done or not said.

When NT participants were asked within the interviews if their partner/family members had prompted conversations for connection to occur, like ASC participants, most gave answers in the negative.

DAWN   *No that's one thing that I noticed that I will*
        say 'You are really frustrating me because ...'
        or 'I am really unhappy because ... ' and he
        never, ever says anything like that. He never
        brings it up.

A few, however, described the occasional circumstance:

SOPHIE   *I think most of the time that he prompts*
         conversation is when the response or decision
         is directly affecting him. For example, the
         ever so common, 'What do you want to do
         for dinner' conversation.

Guiding and Directing Conversations

Most NT participants reported that, in their attempt to gain affection and connection, guiding and directing conversations was the primary prompting behaviour, introduced to encourage more interpersonal involvement from their ASC partner/family members. Most testified that they had an expectation that conversation guidance would lead to an increase in affection and connection. Participants with ASC shared that guiding conversation was not something that they did very often, but they spoke about their partner's or family member's conduct in that regard. Terry's comments revealed that he either mentally or physically withdraws, rather than guide a conversation towards discovering meanings:

> *I used to just sort of mentally tune out but what I've learnt to do over the years with Kim is to actually physically remove myself because she will keep coming at me or trying to meet her needs which at the time unless she actually comes out and says it directly, I quite often have no idea what she really means.*

Barry said that he did not have to work out what his wife meant:

> *Yes, but she is not subliminal about that, I mean she is pretty straightforward, you know she doesn't have to drop hints, put it that way. She would tell me straight out.*

NT participants shared that they often directed conversations to receive more interpersonal involvement from their ASC partners/family members, however, since this was often unwanted by those with ASC, success was either intermittent or non-existent. Renee explained that she has taught her husband how to converse with her:

> *He's learnt now … so when he comes home and instead of going straight over there sitting down and watching TV and waiting for tea … If it's all going well, he'll stand there and we'll talk. He'll say to me 'And how was your day dear?' and*

Have They Gone Nuts?

*I'm like 'Oh okay, good.' So, it is, it's about teaching him ...
I've become very aware of those kinds of prompts if you like.*

Sophie described her direct and to the point communication techniques:

> *I will clearly tell him things like, 'I need you to hold me for a bit', 'I am going to kiss you now', 'Will you please say encouraging or loving things to me', etc. I have to be acutely aware of my own needs and then communicate them to him in a very straightforward manner, so he knows what he needs to do ... but usually [he] applies his own needs first – typical Asperger's. He does notice my physical affections and when I am direct in my verbal communication with him. I have taken numerous upper-level communication courses to help understand more about communication and how to apply things to our relationship in order to improve things.*

Dana described how she worked with her son to help him describe his feelings:

> *He tells me now that he's feeling overwhelmed which is really important. I taught him how to self-advocate years ago back when we were doing a lot with his school work and so using words like ... 'Lets define how we feel.' Do we really feel depressed, or is it more a frustration, or you know, what is going on that's making, you know, this frustration happen?*

On the other hand, Georgia lamented the amount of guidance she had to provide:

> *The things that I felt that another adult should just be able to do without me having to tell them, he couldn't do that*

... You feel like you have to guide them even in the very, very simple things. Even right down to picking the kids up from the damn swimming pool, you have to guide them there, and in the end, it becomes like 'I'll just do it myself'. I found I was just taking more and more and more on because it was just easier to not have to try and guide him through the steps and then also be on the receiving end of the shit he would give you when you were trying to help them. You know, you were nagging, or you were doing it in a way that he didn't want ... talking to him, but because he just wasn't listening ... five minutes later you'd just have to repeat ... that's all communication, that's what makes an effective parenting couple.

Conversation Preparation

Most NT participants reported they had to strengthen prompting with extensive communicational effort to overcome the difficulties. This extra communicational groundwork (to plan, formulate and communicate supporting procedures, to implement preparations prior to initiating conversations, to give detailed explanations, and/or to undertake precise organisations of environmental conditions) involved substantial conversation preparations embedded in prompting, guiding and instructing together with relationship management features. This added communicational workload is usually beyond that which is customary within close relationships but was needed in efforts to contend with the lack of participation within conversations, and resultant chain of behaviours that partner/family members with ASC displayed. It meant that it became the custom to use 'instrumental language' (Murphy, 2015; Reiterer, 2018) rather than using 'declarative language' (Murphy, 2015; Wang, 2016). Declarative language is defined as a statement or comment used to share an opinion (e.g. 'I love spaghetti') or problem-solve (e.g. 'We need tape to fix it'). This declarative type of language does not oblige a verbal response. Rather, it invites experience-sharing, and supplies an ideal social framework for conversational interactions. In general, most conversation includes declarative language. Instrumental language on the other hand is speech that requires a particular response, whether that is an answer to a question or following a direction. The aim of using instrumental language is to influence the listener for certain purposes intended by the speaker. For example, to satisfy basic needs, manipulate the environment or accomplish something (e.g. 'I want…' or 'Can you do…?'). It was found that in neurodiverse relationships, NT participants had to use mostly instrumental language in prompting and guiding conversation and to give repeated explicit step-by-step instructions, practically every time they desired interaction, especially emotional interaction. All NT participants reported that they were compelled to carry out extensive explaining, instructing, teaching, training, guiding or advising, in attempts to solve the problem of inattentive and unresponsive interaction as best they could. Since they were often met with resistance, this communicational groundwork set up a blueprint for the approach the participants used to overcome self-protective behaviours or dependency behaviours, and influence some semblance of relating. Whatever the type of preparation method used, or the reason for prompting, the entire group of NT participants reported that they often did not achieve what they intended. Alex described this difficulty with his ASC partner, Mary:

It's hard, it's very, very difficult negotiating, and theoretically she gets herself in a spin about really small things and that's in an organisational sense sometimes. And it's just like 'Well just, all we need to do is dah, dah, dah' and she will go 'Well, why didn't you explain it like that?' And I'm like 'Well sort of in reality you don't need to explain things like that to people.' … There has to be this structure to it, otherwise it is all confusing. And so that's the way it is. Very step-by-step.

Winnie shared her strategy in giving repeated reminders:

If the issues come up … that we need to discuss as a couple, then I will assess the time when it is a 'good time' to set aside time to talk about that and I will warn him about that so that he can prepare … nothing is sprung on him. I will just mention for a few days in advance, you know we need to talk about this, we need to talk about this, we need to talk about this, and then I will say 'Remember I said we need to talk about this, well I think this is a good time to talk about this.' So, there's all that preparatory work so that he has enough time to prepare and there's nothing that … he is hearing for the first time … We have better conversations, and he will sit and participate in a conversation if I do that preparatory work.

Likewise, Haley shared her recipe for success:

I had to censor everything before I actually attempted to tell him something and I had to make sure I worded it so that it didn't come across like I was attacking … I'd either write down some dot points and I made sure that I stuck to them or I would just make sure in my head I had it straight exactly what I need to say to him and I always started with

121

*'I don't want you to react, I want you to listen to what I
have got to say. I don't want your opinion either. I just need
you to listen and then process it and then I will ask you to
make a choice.'*

Georgia reported that her conversation preparation involved
becoming proficient at 'conversational scene setting', being
cautious with the words that she used and intercepting
conversations that go off track:

*I have to precede …'I'm not criticising,' and learning how to
say your sentences in a way that's not threatening to them,
and then if you were to get it wrong then the shit hits the
fan, because you've said it in the wrong way, or with the
wrong tone of voice, and they feel threatened, or they feel
you're criticising them or you're undermining, and it's like
'Oh my God! You're worse than a teenager.'*

Lilly explained that slowing her discussions down worked
for her:

*I try to slow my voice down. I try to give one instruction at
a time. I try to wait for his responses. Sometimes you know
I mess up and start going on the next thing too.*

Ronda also protested the need to prompt her husband
into having conversations with her, and that he remained
dependent on her prompts in all aspects:

*The initiation for entering into any kind of communication
was always me. Conversation starter is always me, and
initiation for calling or Skyping will always be me and he
just waits until I call … I've tested that over the years to*

see if I stop, will he start, and the answer is – no he will not. So, if I don't initiate then there is nothing, and that's in all aspects of our marriage.

Others revealed strategies that they had found worked for them:

GRACE   *Then I work out – how do I say it easily, like in three sentences, because … you have a need to process and blah, blah, blah, but they don't want that, they want concise quick information and a deadline because … when you tell them, they take it literally, so when you go to them, you need to let them know that they have got time, and I am not expecting an answer straight away otherwise it is this 'Oh my god, I'm being confronted.' Straight away 'I've done something wrong. I am in trouble. Da, da, da.' Of course, it is none of that but that's the thing, so I would probably suggest to people that didn't have an as amazing Aspie as I do, probably to write it if it was something that was important.*

ROBYN   *Sometimes we use diagrams and pictures, or I put a whiteboard out there, in the last couple of months, and I draw something on the whiteboard.*

An anonymous NT survey respondent said:

Have to learn skills other than the usual social skills in order to have successful communication with an Aspie.

For example: have to think in advance about how to frame requests in terms of what he would get out of it. Have to think prior to raising issues about how to say things in a way that he will receive them. Have to be more rational and not emotive at all. As soon as any emotion is involved, he shuts down. So spontaneous discussions don't happen.

In Summary

To compensate for their difficulties, most ASC participants attempted to bypass the majority of interpersonal conversations by resorting to various avoidance behaviours, such as unresponsiveness, conversation avoidance, walking away and not asking interpersonal questions. These behaviours often resulted in misinterpreting the actions of others and forming inaccurate assumptions based on what they observed. While the intended outcome of these avoidance behaviours was to cope with their inabilities, and consequently, avoid emotional conversation, an often-unintended outcome was that these strategies became triggers for their NT partner and family members to compensate. Through prompting, guiding and directing, and planning conversations, the compensatory behaviours used by NT participants were intended to overturn the compensatory behaviours of their ASC partner and family members. A tug-of-war between the two distinct compensatory behaviours of each, often resulted.

Thus, most conversations seeking affection, connectedness and personal communication became an ongoing pattern of contrasting needs and follow-on communication problems. These problems influenced a systematic strengthening of each approach, by each person. The resulting increases in unresponsive and avoidant behaviour led to increases in prompting and extra communicational work. An ongoing pattern formed due to the stability of the distinct and differing abilities, needs and viewpoints of each on how to solve rising problems, combined with the escalation of alternating irreconcilable forces that consisted of contrasting needs, compensatory strategies and tactics to solve the resulting problems. The result of this ongoing pattern is discussed in the next chapter.

7

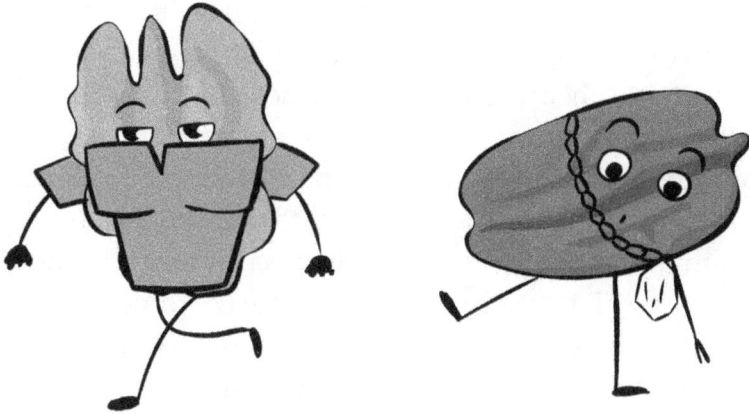

A Permanent Millstone

Have They Gone Nuts?

**'The limits of my language mean
the limits of my world.'**
Ludwig Wittgenstein

A Catch 22

Regarding prompting, a 'catch 22'[2] occurs from the partial effectiveness of the prompting strategy. Given that intermittent schedules of reinforcement are very resistant to extinction (Lerman et al., 1996), the partial effectiveness of prompting became influential in intensifying the level of prompting over time. A requirement to manage relationships through prompting caused an imbalance in the relationship, and when NT participants endeavoured to correct this imbalance, the reverse was found to occur. As participants with ASC continued to depend on prompts, paradoxically, prompting was required to end prompting. So, rather than being released from an obligation to prompt, NT participants had to increase it. Consequently, prompting became the main way that most relationship matters took place.

Thus, contrasting needs led to contrasting compensatory strategies which influenced a systematic strengthening of each approach, by each person. More unresponsive and avoidant behaviour kept pace with more prompting and its extra communicational work. Yet, interaction incompatibilities remained. Unresponsive and avoidant behaviour remained. Due to the permanency of the distinct and differing abilities, needs and viewpoints on how to solve rising problems,

---

[2] A paradoxical situation from which an individual cannot escape (Heller, 1961)

and the escalation of alternating irreconcilable forces, an ongoing pattern formed in most conversations on affection, connectedness and personal communication.

Although the different requirements for emotional, personal and meaningful conversations were the reasons for the diametrically opposed behaviours of each, the combination of prompting behaviour, conversation avoidance, unresponsiveness to and/or withdrawal from affectionate communications, and the inability to discuss problems and deal with resulting conflicts, were all circumstances that not only triggered prompting, but also increased the intensity of prompting behaviours of NT participants.

Walking Away

Many ASC partner/family members showed a propensity to physically remove themselves to avoid conversations. Tracy (NT) described how James (ASC) would leave in the middle of conversations:

> I feel like I am trying to communicate with a robot that has been programmed to speak as little as possible. James can go for weeks without any form of communication apart from 'I'm going to town', 'See you later', 'What time do the girls come home?', 'Bye.' He has no need for more … It has happened SO often that he goes downstairs right in the middle of a conversation. He just leaves the room, he needs to go out, he needs to do something down there, he needs to be elsewhere … And I'm left calling 'COME BACK! I haven't finished! How can I talk to you when you are in another room?' Or I follow him downstairs and try to continue talking. But

when he goes elsewhere, it also means that he is not willing to continue the conversation, so there is not much point in pursuing him.

Jim (ASC) gave a candid account of how his interaction difficulties impacted on him, preferring to walk away to solve the situation:

Just shut up and walk away, and of course, that makes it worse because Dianne wants a good working relationship in regard to communication. Like I would have a situation where I tried to express how I feel, and before I can, because I've got to stop and think about it, and I've got to go round corners and have to go a long way around to get to my point. Well sorry Dianne doesn't, Dianne has got to get to the point straight away … Well I'm not capable of doing it … whereas Dianne is just 'If you've got something to say, say it' yeah, well I'm not as blunt as you are sometimes. But it makes it extremely difficult.

On the other hand, Dianne (NT) shared how Jim frequently avoided relating to her, only choosing to communicate when in the company of others, or else redirecting the conversation:

He won't talk about it when we are on our own, but he will express it when we are with a group cause he knows that I won't respond when we are in a group, because it is not appropriate. So, he is smart to do that. … So, redirects it, or takes something else somewhere else that is not even to do with what the issue is because he probably doesn't want to deal with it, or he has been told the truth. Can't deal well with the truth, and the facts.

Alternatively, Malcolm said that awareness of his diagnosis and working to understand the differences improved his abilities to relate to his family. Even though there were still times when he didn't want to relate to his NT partner and avoid the situation, avoidance occurred to a lesser degree. He described that his avoidance strategies included running away and hiding in a cupboard or else putting his 'walls' up (blocking interaction and connection):

> *Oh, I will go and hide in my cupboard. I have got a cupboard that I go into. If I get really frustrated … I would just explode, verbally. Not angrily but I will just tumble out all this crap, which is not really relevant telling people off, or Grace in this case, just blah, blah, blah, and then I will go and hide in my cupboard … Probably go and sulk for a couple of days. Just be really quiet and I would probably ignore Grace, which I am doing less and less, cause I'm aware that it is not supportive behaviour. It's destructive … So we had the worst times then and of course it deteriorated because the more she wanted to reach out, the more I would run away … when my walls are up, no-one is getting anywhere near me, no matter what they say, and no matter how loving Grace is … I mean, the family knows now. My oldest daughter will just tell me 'Dad, just go to your cupboard.' Or she says, one of the other things 'Dad, just relax. Just relax.'*

Grace, Malcolm's NT partner described the difference understanding can make to their communication. She drew comparisons between what her relationship was like before Malcolm's Asperger diagnosis to after the diagnosis:

> *I have developed my sense of self because there are certain parts of the Aspergersness that really trigger, like a human*

reaction in people. If you're misunderstood, you want to correct it straight away. And I remember the early stages, I would see that he was upset by something, but of course, you never know what it is and so … I would want to fix it there and then … before we knew about Asperger's. I soon learnt that is not the way to do it. But even now there is sometimes, if a Matilda is really bad, or it comes across suddenly and, Malcolm's got it down pat. Like he hardly has them. It's like six or eight months and he'll have a Matilda. And it used to be, when we were first started, a Matilda could last two or three days, you know, just this stillness and non-communication and whatever, and now really, he is so aware … he just recognises it so there's no actual impact on the family and then when he has a real Matilda, it is very brief. You know, and it's nothing aggressive or horrible or, a Matilda is just 'he is freaked out about something, and he just wants to retreat'. Yeah, so there's no abuse, or there's nothing external going on. I suppose, a healthy human might think it's abusive that your partner can't communicate but I think if you have love and understanding because you straight away want to go into 'what's wrong with me' or 'what did I do to make that happen' and really, it's got nothing to do with you … The biggest struggle I had early stages … was that need to be right or heard … 'it is not what I meant' or 'I need you to understand what I meant', and I just don't do that anymore.

Some NT participants described other behaviours that their ASC partners/family members used to avoid conversations:

LUCY   *If I want to talk about a specific subject …*
            he's not terribly interested in hearing this.

'Yep, yep, yep, yep' he has this habit of saying back all the time, in other words 'Oh shut up I don't want to listen to you.' And I'll say 'Look really I'd like to talk to you about this,' but if he doesn't want to talk about it, he doesn't want to talk about it and ... he does his best to shut me down and I've since realised that if that's the case I've got to go and have a communication session with my friends because we can communicate and we do have other similar opinions or differing opinions and we'll discuss it and debate it and stuff like that but having a debate with him is, you just couldn't do it, no way.

FIONA   *I get frustrated because I'm explaining the same thing and being corrected on the way I described it. Although William tells me that he is only reconfirming, but it is not the way he is wording it. I feel frustrated. I feel angry. I feel defeated.*

Constructing Roadblocks

Several comments from participants with ASC showed that they understood that their unresponsiveness to their partner/family members' prompts limited the fulfilment of intended outcomes. Mark confirmed that he understood how his NT partner wanted him to respond to her. However, he revealed that he often shut down during their interactions:

Ah, she will quite often try and get me to respond in the way that she wants me to respond, so she will keep at me … she will often say things that she knows that will get a response through trying to hurt me, name-calling, that sort of thing, she may resort to. Recently she has admitted that she does actually actively do that to try and get a response out of me, because when that sort of thing happens, I start shutting down. So, there's going to be no visible response from me, no emotional response, which apparently frustrates the crap out of her.

On the other hand, some mentioned that a lack of responsiveness had the potential to avert some prompting. Sandra's words gave that impression:

He definitely tries to prompt it … because I'm not always positively responding back … he doesn't really try as much as he used to.

The lack of ability to relate, work through misunderstandings and make progress toward resolutions led to much conflict and distress. Jim expressed the sentiment of many participants with ASC:

She will make a comment that 'You don't listen to me or anything like that' but neither does she listen to me, so it makes it a bit hard, we are trying to interact, we are either yelling, or she doesn't listen, where she will explain, 'Well there is a typical example of your behaviour', but she doesn't see her behaviour exactly the same, and of course, she doesn't believe that her behaviour is anything different to what it has been … because I am the way I am …

However, many NT participants felt that unresponsiveness and the effort it took to gain a response was one of the most demanding things to deal with in their relationship. Tracy shared her frustrations behind the effort to gain a response:

I have to ask so many questions just to get a very basic piece of information ... I have told him time and time again that I am no wiser after one of his answers than before I asked the question.

She lamented the realisation that no matter the amount of effort, there was still an ongoing lack of emotional connection:

I get the impression that for him, a satisfactory conclusion would be me saying yes to everything he says and not having a mind of my own. He does not seem to understand that it means BOTH of us have to make concessions and take a step towards each other. Of course, a lot of the time our expectations and needs are just so different that he does not see why I should need such and such. Like when I tried to explain to him that I felt lonely, and he told me he would go away for a few weeks so I would understand what 'lonely' meant. He did not understand that one could feel lonely when the other was physically present. He does not understand what needs to happen between two people so there is no loneliness, what his wife needs so that she feels like a wife, that being WITH someone is not just physical presence. I do not think there is anyone who could tell me they have actually felt WITH James with an emotional connection. I now realise that for years and years I thought there was some emotional connection, wondered about the problems, but in fact there was not.

Have They Gone Nuts?

Grace described some of the responsiveness differences between her and Malcolm:

> *When you are having a discussion, 'Like what do you think about this?' I would love him to be able to just respond to me. And sometimes he knows that, and he tries, but really what it needs to be is 'Hi, I want to talk to you about this. This is my view. Go and have a think about it and get back to me when you want to.' So again, that's like that humanness of having something shared. You don't have that ... he says to me 'Just give me the information. I will sit with that information' ... their inward processes are not like our outward processes. They just pull out the facts ... It's all about minus emotion, but the funny thing is they have so much emotion inside themselves ... They don't express it to you, but it is massive in here. They are so sensitive ... if you make a statement 'Can you do this?' and their reaction is 'Oh the world is coming to an end. You hate me. I have stuffed up.' I mean that is such an emotive thing going on.*

Dana's account revealed variations in responsiveness between her ASC ex-partner and her ASC son:

> *Miles seems to be really needy about me, and always has been ... If I call him or if I send him a note, he responds immediately ... He can't wait to talk to me. Jay is a little bit less inclined to do that ... He likes to be really demonstrative about not responding.*

However, Derek (NT) expressed how he tired of Cora's dependence on his social support which made him retreat from her:

Oh, it means that I'm sort of ah … it is a point of friction … she becomes more needing my attention and I back away more. So, I'm looking for space and she is looking for more attention so that ends up being a bit of a negative cycle cause the more she, you know paws at me, the more I pull away and so it can get into a bit of a downward spiral.

Enclosed in Armour

Opting not to discuss problems, most ASC participants openly commented on their various defensive, unresponsive and avoidant behaviours:

WALLY *Back out, leave the room … It just allows me to not become so emotionally overwhelmed.*

MURRAY *It's very easy to get defensive … if it goes from a discussion to more an accusation of what you're doing wrong, then that's where I probably don't want to talk about it.*

MARY *I can come across as very caustic and critical sometimes, because, and it's not because I think that person has necessarily done the wrong thing, it's because they are not doing it the way that I asked them to. It comes back to am I being heard properly.*

SANDRA *I get more uncomfortable in a conversation that's going to go on and on about something negative, especially when a lot of times it's two opposing sides of something so in my eyes*

> *we're not going to get to any kind of result you know if we're on two different sides of the situation so to me I'm like let's just let it go and move on to something else.*

BARRY   *If I had done something silly and then she will have a go at me and then I will think, yeah okay, it is done. What can I do about it? Let's just close it now. Doesn't make any difference discussing it.*

Most NT participants described that they dealt with their partner/family members unresponsive and avoidant behaviours through learning to become very direct, giving explicit instructions and increasing their prompting practices.

MIA   *The way I talk about my needs and the way that I request some responses from him is very direct ... Previously, I wasn't ... That was before he had the diagnosis, and we had the knowledge of the way he thinks and functions and our differences.*

GEORGIA   *When I ask him something, don't expect an answer straight away, just give him the time to process and sometimes you have to actually prod and give him clues.*

Most NT participants were aware that the unresponsiveness toward them often came from a lack of awareness, which was unintentional. They revealed that they were willing to give support in achieving more awareness and communicational responsiveness. However, the rigid thinking of their ASC partner/family members prevented improved communication and blocked the NT participants' abilities to improve the communication from their position. Not only did difficulties with solving problems and working together create a need for many NT participants to be direct and prompt for resolutions, but the resistance they also faced, set up a sense of loneliness and a loss of a desired 'sense of togetherness' in shared activities. Katy shared how this was the case for her on both accounts:

> I got some very useful tips from the clinician; what I do is I say when something is unacceptable, and I just leave it at that … If he doesn't want to do something he just doesn't do it. You cannot force him to do anything he doesn't want to do. And I mean this is one of the lonely spots in our relationship, is that he will be motivated to do something that he wants to do, but for me to ask him to do something, it's like I have asked him to pin himself to a cross. It is just so resistive, and he might do it eventually, after months and months of me asking, but he will do it with such foul temper that it is almost a waste of me getting anything done. And it never gets finished. He never finishes anything that he doesn't want to do.

Fiona described how communication often came to a halt due to this rigidity:

> He tells me 'No that's not what all this is about.' He talks over the top of me. And I just finished up telling him to shut up and walk away … it's just like hitting your head against a brick wall all the time.

Renee revealed that problem-solving in her household became a function of pre-planning, followed by prompts that included lists and instructions:

> *I've learnt that problems don't get solved in our relationship by talking about them, they get solved by me thinking about them, thinking through and then going with him 'Right this is what we need to do,' which takes me back to me being the boss ... which in most relationships that is not how you do things but he was just absolutely okay with that, it was like 'Oh okay then.'*

An anonymous comment from an ASC survey respondent revealed a common perspective of those with ASC towards those who are NT:

> *I always seem to say and do the wrong thing. Because I have an ASD and mental health diagnosis, my husband believes he is therefore always right about everything. Whenever I try to address something, he has done or said which has hurt me, I am seen as acting irrationally or misrepresenting or distorting things. He often outright does not believe something I've said, or has been said or done to me, unless he was a witness. I feel like, he thinks I'm a liar. Because he has no diagnosis, therefore 100% of the time, he is right. I'm so tired of the fighting which never resolves things, as he won't change behaviour or apologise for hurting me (despite me making efforts to change everything about my personality and apologising). I've asked him to let me move out or let me die.*

Alternatively, a comment from an NT survey respondent expressed a common perspective of those who are NT towards those with ASC:

A Permanent Millstone

My sister is so sweet and fun when she wants to actually talk but otherwise is oblivious to the fact that we exist and would like some communication. She seems not to need her family's interaction believing it is interference more than genuine interest.

Taken Hostage

Most involved in a neurodiverse relationship were found to be taken hostage by their differences. No matter what the occasion, circumstance or the rationalisation, the standpoint appeared to be the same for both groups of participants. Participants with ASC merely complied when prompted or avoided the prompts and NT participants continued to prompt for what they needed. Each displayed the notion that if the other would simply concede, all would be well. Most participants with ASC described a need for emotional recovery to be undertaken alone. However, they showed unawareness that this self-protective behaviour ensnared them in the prompting behaviour of their NT partner/family members in the first place, and refusal to implement the behaviour prompted ensnared them in it even more:

MALCOLM *If Grace talks to me, if I take it personally, … I don't say anything, but she wants to converse, but I don't have that ability. I can't. What you mean you want to talk about this? I'm right and you're wrong. You're doing your thing, there is nothing to talk about and then I run away … Like she will say 'Can you take out the rubbish?' And I will hear 'I haven't done the rubbish. I haven't taken it out all week.*

I have failed in taking out the rubbish. Why haven't I done it properly?' You know I have to go through that process before I realise that she is just asking me to take out the rubbish. Or she is trying to talk to me about an aspect of our relationship, that's what I hear is noise and yelling and confusion, so I have to go away and process it. And then she will follow me and will talk more, and it is like 'No, no, no, no!'

SAMUEL   *After the diagnosis I became more stand-offish ... in knowing that I'm wired differently and in order to act normally is a real strain. I'd rather just save my energy and enjoy myself doing what I want.*

TERRY   *Well I tend to back off and sort of zone out ... I'm noticing that I do tend to withdraw a lot, in those sorts of situations.*

TOM   *Sometimes difficult conversations cause me to feel attacked and I respond defensively and sometimes angrily ... I tell him I don't want to talk about it anymore.*

However, Max shared a different perspective:

You know if you don't have the humility to respond to your external suggestions you don't improve ... If you're not prepared to be humble to some extent then whether you're on the spectrum or whether you're neurotypical the lack of humility will inevitably affect the relationship ... but I think

to some extent you also have to go to a place where you're
not comfortable.

Most NT participants reported that they tried to accommodate their ASC partner or family member's differences, especially after a diagnosis. Yet, they needed to do what they needed to do. To talk through times of upset and problems was a driving force, of which prompting became a standard feature. However, trying to untangle the resulting conflict, often became the cause of more conflict:

MAGGIE   *He's happy with no or very little connection,*
          he's quite content with it. So yeah, I'm not …
          I was feeling very unloved, very uncared for
          and he was shutting down to every strategy,
          everything I was trying to do to help our
          relationship and get a connection with him
          and so he ended up going into a meltdown, is
          what I think, and that's when he packed up
          and he left because he was so stressed because I
          was pushing because I wanted the connection.

QUINN   *I would start a conversation in bed and he*
          would never say anything and I would just
          have to turn around and go to sleep, because
          20/30 minutes would go by and it was that
          silence … and I told him …'I can't handle
          this. I cannot do this anymore.' I said, 'So
          if I ask you something you better have an
          answer for it, or come up with one, because
          it's just very painful to me.' And I told him
          'I'm not willing to do that anymore, so I
          think I've already bent all that I can, I can't

adjust myself anymore', so those are our conversations, very difficult.

KATY   *I always try and set the scene. Every time I talk to him about any issue that I know it is going to be difficult, I try and set the scene, but 99.9% of the time it will backfire ... That's when he really does a retreat, and he will even get up and walk away from me while I'm talking.*

FIONA   *It depends how much energy I have on the day, whether to humour him into doing it, but lately that hasn't been possible because he has been so antagonistic towards me. Before he got the diagnosis, I could humour him into almost anything that needed doing.*

Many NT participants also described the difficulties of dealing with the full-scale meltdowns that can occur during difficult conversations. When Laura was asked if she talked about difficulties in her relationship with her partner, she answered that *'it caused a meltdown'*. And when asked how he responds, she said *'raging, followed by both flight but also appeasing. No deeper mutual understanding'*.

Dawn also mentioned that difficult discussions often strengthen into rage:

I noticed when in heated discussion ... if he is in an argument with anybody else, he will win the argument, he is very, very, very good at arguing, (sigh). When he is in an argument with me, he loses the plot really quickly. He loses his temper

... He doesn't become abusive or anything like that ... he just boils over very quickly, and I have always observed that, it's like that's weird why ... I can stay in control, and for me it's a heated discussion, he has lost the plot, he's just raging, and can't, so angry, that's weird because he doesn't get like that with anybody else.

Diana described how a meltdown can get quite serious:

He just gets frustrated and gets worked up to such a degree that he then lashes out and is violent and then he's sorry and remorseful and whatever else afterward but he doesn't seem to completely understand that that's not a sign of affection and that he's saying he loves me but then that sort of thing is happening so yeah, it's just I suppose for him, he doesn't seem to, he can't seem to wrap his head around it.

Whereas Lucy said:

Well, I don't live with him and never have in fact. I ran scared when he wanted me to go and live with him because I find him very controlling. They hate getting out of their comfort zone. They're regimented and I realised that his home was never going to be my home. He had to have everything of his in this place and so on and so forth, so I backed out of that, and it was so fortunate that I did because I know it wouldn't have worked. So, I'm one of the lucky ones, I guess. When I meet all of the other people at the group that I attend and they're all married, well some of them have now separated, I think I really am lucky because when he starts, I can just say, 'Look I've got to go home now.' And that's the way I've handled it since I found out.

In Summary

Commonly, communication (both verbal and non-verbal) is the very means used to improve interpersonal interaction or resolve differences of opinion. However, if the very processes used to achieve understanding or resolve differences increases misunderstanding and difficulties, constructing competent interaction becomes almost impossible, and the means by which understanding and commonality may be achieved also becomes almost impossible. As a result of these perpetual problems the majority of ASC participants became frustrated, anxious, distressed and confused, due to their partner/family members' propensity to want to discuss problems. These reactions, some ASC participants confirmed, were frequently due to a lack of understanding of how to fix any communication problems with their partner/family members or how to respond to resultant distress. Many ASC participants confided they felt incapable of communicating in a way that was required of them, and these circumstances led them to become overwhelmed. Some indicated that they relied on the help of their partner/family members. Others, however, resented this help, preferring to withdraw rather than address the problem. Either way, rather than working on the cause of the problem themselves, ASC participants tended to allow their partner/family members to continue to attempt solutions on their own and, in the process, become dependent on the prompts delivered to them, or else avoid the prompts given through self-protective means.

Although the success of prompting was an on-again off-again occurrence, the unpredictability between avoidance behaviour and random dependency on prompts was found to be the catalyst that set in motion a process of oscillation between prompting on the part of the NT participants and response and/or avoidance on the part of their partner/family members with ASC. It was this process of oscillation, combined with conversation inabilities and anxieties, which worked to increase the self-protective behaviours displayed by those with ASC. These processes also worked to increase the conversational behaviours displayed by those who are NT. When taken together, a complex system of circular conversations was established within these relationships, and these cycling difficulties are discussed in the next chapter.

8

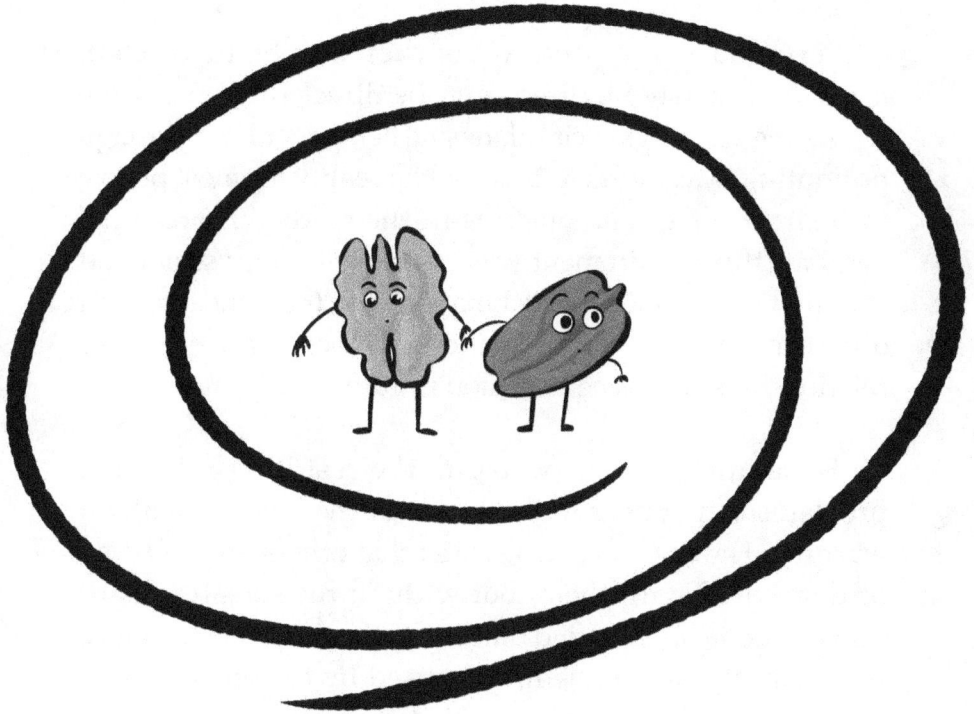

The Cycle Ensnares

Have They Gone Nuts?

**'All problems exist in the
absence of a good conversation.'**
Thomas Leonard

An Unrelenting Cycle

Perpetually required to instruct, and be instructed, teach, and be taught, direct, and be directed, all the while regulating all things social alongside being regulated through prompting, was found to become the reality for most people in neurodiverse relationships in the study. Whereas the basis for this requirement was traceable to poor social and communication skills in combination with the difficulties and differences discussed, the experience of these matters in close relationships can place enormous strain on all concerned.

For adults on the spectrum, the resulting relational problems can appear to come 'out of the blue' or without warning. Having some awareness that others are confused or displeased with them, but without the social skills or conversational tools to find out why and correct their conduct, they may see the problems as caused by the other person. Without the ability to 'connect the dots' or see the patterns in their own social conduct or speech, as explanations for their dilemma, they may feel unjustly accused. If they realise they are making mistakes, often during a sequence of behavioural and language choice errors, it can be too late for them to repair a deteriorated social situation. The result is continuous misunderstandings, misinterpretations and social interaction mistakes. In contrast, for NT adults, the opportunities that they were looking to communicate, connect, express love, and give and receive emotional support through social reciprocity in their relationships was prevented by these difficulties and differences, and attempts to put matters right were likewise prevented.

Thus, the diametrically opposed needs and abilities of people within neurodiverse relationships was found to activate endless cycles of unsolvable communication difficulties and differences between them. The constant interplay between the lack of communicational abilities, accompanied with subsequent stonewalling tactics to avoid communicating on the part of those with ASC, when combined with the prompting that NT participants introduced to gain interaction and connection, became a communication roundabout full of confusion and conflict for most participants in these studies. This interplay triggered the prompt dependency phenomenon while also maintaining it. When one intensified so did the other. Efforts by NT participants to overcome unresponsive and avoidant behaviours were met with either compliance merely when prompted, or else an often-unyielding resistance on the part of their ASC partner/family members. Self-reliant initiation of the behaviour prompted did not materialise. Most NT participants revealed that they became embedded in trying to explain, talk, prompt and instruct to achieve solutions to communication problems with their partner/family members with ASC. However, in the face of strong resistance and the presence of persistent disharmony within communications, most NT participants reported an experience of built-up resentment toward their partner/family members with ASC. Alongside this, the efforts of those with ASC to avoid unwanted interaction were also met with an often-unyielding resistance through prompting. Thus, a communication cycle, of which prompting with dependency and/or avoidance of prompts played corresponding functions; coping with the escalating difficulties and trying to achieve opposing needs. The twofold impact of imparting prompts on the one hand and prompt dependency/avoidance on the other were shown to have a negative influence on these relationships. Some ASC participants discussed the unresolvable nature of their cyclic disagreements. Stella described how constant and unresolvable their circular conversations were:

> We raise the same topics over and over again – child rearing, money and chores and it seems that we never reach a final conclusion.

Terry outlined the escalating nature of some of his cyclic types of conversations:

> I have one point of view and she has another one. Whether it's one person is right or wrong or whether it's a communication misunderstanding again we get this sort of 'ratcheting up' scenario that seems to happen.

Sandra shared the futility to being caught in the cycle:

> I'm saying the same thing over and over because I don't have anything more to maybe say in this situation, except you know just saying over and over my side of it so it kind of is a bit redundant to me, and if I don't see it going anywhere it just becomes like I don't know what else to say.

Rachelle (ASC) and Ryan (NT), one of the couples involved in the study, also felt that they could not progress pass a certain point, therefore they had both given up:

RACHELLE *Because what annoys us about each other …*
we're beyond the point of bothering to fix them
and to try to not do that thing anymore.

RYAN *I'm not sure that going deeper into a*
conversation would actually resolve anything.
We go as deep as we need to go and either
there is going to be a resolution or not going
to be a resolution. If there is not going to be a
resolution there's going to be an argument and
a fight and I don't tend to want to go in that
territory myself … she can get quite worked
up over a decision that is not going her way
… She has been known to throw things at me
in the past too, so I don't tend to want to go
into that territory.

All NT participants interviewed, repeatedly mentioned how difficult it was to live with the unproductive circular characteristics to most of their conversations. Rae lamented the frustration and confusion that resulted:

And you go round and round the mountain and still don't
come up with an answer … but I mean they just tip you over
the edge with the frustration and the annoyance and I just
think 'why is this so hard?' I can talk, have a conversation
with anybody else and everybody else can understand me
… You just get so confused when I try to talk … I lay it all
out there you, still … are going round and round in circles.
People have got no idea, have they?

Haley described how the progress of time had only made the circumstances worse:

Have They Gone Nuts?

*[We] couldn't get off the merry-go-round and ended up …
in a screaming match … I used to try and reason, like as
a normal person would … I would listen to what he was
saying, and he would just get angrier and angrier because
… in his eyes, I wasn't listening to him. That's the way that
he has seen it … and they just keep repeating themselves
over and over, 'You don't understand how I feel, you know,
you don't know how I feel.' Yes, I do understand because
you have told me. In the end … I would just either say …
'I'm just not talking about this anymore' because you're not
getting anywhere … Because it had to stop, because it was
just going on and on in circles and unless I got really sucked
in on this merry-go-round … I would just say I'm not, I'm
over this, it is finished … I'm not doing this anymore.*

Similarly, Dawn described how circular conversations had
not improved over their many years together:

*I would wonder why we kept coming back in this cycle.
Because it was never getting anywhere. Why was I never
getting anywhere? … so, yeah I guess I'm the one that
has pushed for better communication and instigate the
reconnecting after we have had a squabble … I have said
'we need to improve communication', and we never do, and
if we do, it's because I had instigated it and I have learned
not to assume, I've learned to ask, and sometimes I get a
stroppy, surly 12-year-old teenager answer and sometimes
I get a normal answer … I don't think it has improved over
the years … we go round and round, or I go round and
round about that.*

Shirley also described 'endless cycles' of miscommunication:

154

The Cycle Ensnares

So many of our arguments ... are based on misunderstandings and we just keep getting into a cycle of 'but I didn't mean that, I meant this', 'well that's not how I took it, I felt this' and it just keeps going around and around and the arguments ... tend to be of a cyclic nature ... about the same things so ... we get stuck in these endless cycles of the same kind of arguments.

Sabrina expressed it as a 'dog chasing its tail' that they could not escape:

We just end up ... it's the dog chasing its tail ... when it's about us and our relationship it's just a circle that we can't get out of.

Georgia explained how the circular conversations became mind-bending arguments that made her question her sanity:

Conversations with regard to say the children and trying to explain to him what their needs are as children and not expect them to understand his Asperger's, not at this point anyway, not at this age and that is a circular conversation and it goes round and it goes round ... and it will end up with him blaming me or just disagreeing ... and so that's another example of this huge circular conversation over a very important issue ... first of all it was denial, and then it was like let's go off on a tangent, let's deflect and then it's throw it back at her, that well really it's your fault anyway and you're being the cruel one here ... I ended up feeling like ... I'm being unreasonable or am I not understanding this and I had to go and seek, talk to my girlfriends about it to say 'Am I crazy?' ... Should I be more understanding or was he wrong? ... it was one of those conversations that make you question your sanity and whether you're behaving right and whether your actions are right and you kind of know inside yourself that what you're doing is right because it feels right that your human reaction is right, but they're telling you it's wrong to behave that way and that you're in the wrong here. 'You don't understand what's going on. You should be the bigger person.' ... No. And if you're having, and it's not just one conversation a day, it's multiple conversations every day on every level whether it be just, take the trash out and all of a sudden, you're a witch and you're terrible for asking him to take the trash out, to much bigger issues like the one I just explained, even the little things are made complicated.

The Cycle Captures

A complex system of circular conversations was found to emerge from the conflict of one needing to keep matters unchanged, while the other needing to change those same matters. Captured by the cycle, Fiona (NT) illustrated the often-seen relationship between the prompting behaviours triggering aggression in response:

Every time there is no, there's no memory of the last time that was done. Everything is new every day. Every day! ... Draining and frustrating. And sometimes I just say 'You drive me crazy. Absolutely crazy.' I used to yell it at him. Now I just say it. Because it is not helping my health ... I'm trying to change the way I interact with him, but what I'm finding is it's not changing because he's bringing in new behaviours that keeps us in that conflict situation. And that's why I hope someone can get through to him because I can't. Can't, and I don't want to stay in that conflict. I want to move on. Life's too short ... I get frustrated because I'm explaining the same thing and being corrected on the way I described it ... Oh, a lot of anger which I can't internalise anymore. I punched the wall the other night, instead of punching him. That's got to stop ... Shame. I can't believe that I would treat someone I love in that manner ... I never ever thought. I did hit him once. He hit me back. I don't blame him. It is unacceptable behaviour from one human being to another. I don't believe I've been reduced to reacting in that manner.

Thus, the need for reciprocal interaction (NT participant) and the need to avoid reciprocal interaction (ASC participant) were the common threads that kept prompt dependency/ avoidance cycling between the two and that triggered the prompt dependency phenomenon. This cycling entangled communication system was found to become the main way of relating in neurodiverse relationships.

Most NT participants acknowledged that they struggled with many negative consequences from the effort involved in dealing with the need to continually prompt for interaction and connection, while also prompting to repair misunderstandings and key areas of conflict. The negative consequences were especially felt when the self-protective behaviours of their ASC partner/family members undermined their efforts to try to improve the situation. In view of that, the amount of conversational effort they had to undertake, was the product of erroneous interactions that they attempted to remedy. The remedy, however, also negatively affected them since their ASC partner or family member's lack of awareness often triggered many other negative behaviours. Haley said as much:

I had to censor everything before I actually attempted to tell him something. And I had to make sure I worded it so that it didn't come across like I was attacking them or that it was offensive and then I had to make sure that when he got the whole gist of it that he didn't turn it into a big thing about him, because it always went back to him. Every conversation. Didn't matter what I spoke about or what we were trying to discuss it always went back to him, you know. 'I know that I've been an arse, and I know I've done this, and it is all my fault.' That is what the conversation always went back to.

On the other hand, Sabrina illustrated that her partner went the other way, blaming her:

Well in the beginning I would just complain and then he would say 'You're criticising me' and I said, 'I'm not criticising, I am just stating the facts' and I said, 'What approach do you suggest? What should I say?' I mean you really kind of run out of ways to clean it up, so to speak, when you're just stating the facts … so what ends up happening is that he will turn it back on me, and tell me 'Oh it's all about you, it's all about you' … which is just bizarre.

Sophie's method was to keep questioning to keep conversations from moving into negative territory:

I also have to be acutely aware of how he is interpreting my message, so he doesn't take it as a negative. Because AS men are more apt to hear criticism in things, even when there is none. I have to ask him what he heard, or how he feels, to see if he interpreted the message the way I intended. He is also not shy about communicating with me his emotional state, so I know what and how to communicate with him. He normally responds quite well.

For similar reasons, Quinn had decided not to bring anything up anymore:

It got to a point where it almost felt like it was walking on eggshells, because every time I would talk to him he would get so defensive. I just kind of got tired of not getting anywhere and just being accused … it's just something that happened within me I guess, another defence mechanism, I just … wasn't bringing anything up anymore because I just didn't feel that it was worth it.

Diana said that prompting was seen as nagging, but prompting was the only way to make things happen:

I think sometimes that can be a little bit blurred for him and one problem is because he does need prompting with a lot of things. He takes that as nagging. It gets kind of blurred and you're kind of always catching your tail pretty much, just chasing after your tail, he doesn't seem to, well he wants to help, he says you're not helping me, so you're helping him, but then you're nagging. So yeah, it is a catch 22 pretty much all of the time.

Georgia shared her husband's description of his struggles:

My husband did say … prior to his diagnosis, 'Sometimes when we have conversations … you can move so fast and switch so quickly and … I cannot keep up. The speed which you get from things and make connections … I'm left lagging behind. By the time I've processed one thing that you've said

159

and felt the emotion that's connected with that one thing that you've said, you've already moved on to the next thing.'

Then she added:

Because that's the way we are, it's so natural. There is no thought for us. It's just instinctual. It just comes, whereas he has to hear it, think it, process it, then feel it, then process it, think it, and then respond … Sometimes when you're talking to them, they just go quiet. You ask them and you're like – respond; and they don't respond! And I'm thinking that must be what they're doing, they're thinking, and they're processing, and they're trying to understand what it is you said, and that was one thing that I learnt to do that when I am talking … is to try and slow down. And that was one thing his counsellor said sometimes, you know, you need to say the words, or give him clues, just to help him along the way, how sometimes you do with kids, if they can't find the word. They're learning a language and they can't find the word, so you have to label it for them and then they can make a sentence. That's almost sometimes like what it's like, having a conversation with him but that's draining.

Like Georgia, Dianne shared her frustrations and drew attention to the lack of words, the lack of emotion, and the unresponsiveness that she experienced:

I know that my ranting and raving only makes that worse, and he withdraws all the more because I guess he hasn't got the words. But he doesn't show anything, like there is no emotion. Like not even a touch or a hug, or a 'it will be okay', or a recognition even that you are hurting, even though it's got to be obvious that you are.

Then she shared her dismay at how the progression of time had not resolved the situation:

> *But now he withdraws because I just nowadays have the total wrong, wrong tactic. I probably did years ago, would sit and 'Well tell me and talk to me' and I would get a blank sort of inane sort of stare, and I have often had things like, 'Well I don't really know' and I actually believe that he doesn't. I think that's part of the frustration. I don't know, but I figure at 57 there has got to be somewhere along the line you've got to know something. Over 35 years if you still don't know, something is just not working.*

On the other hand, Jim, (ASC) Dianne's husband, illustrated his lack of awareness:

> *I have had situations where I would be sitting on a chair, she would be on the floor bawling her eyes out and say, 'Why can't you understand?' And I would say 'Understand what?' And this is the point, so to be fair on that question, well in a lot of instances I didn't really know whether things were right or wrong, so it makes it a bit hard.*

The difficulties that ASC participants experienced with communication and with its resulting series of behaviours were found to precede a great deal of confusion for them. Often, this confusion surfaced as another reason to become self-protective. The demand to communicate, with ever-present evidence of their NT partner or family member's distress at their lack of ability to communicate appeared to be one of the main motives for self-protective reasoning and resulting self-protective behaviour. Regularly, angry outbursts afforded a means to withdraw from communicating.

Regardless of whether ASC partners/family members were initially confused by the difficulties, or wanting to avoid all forms of communication altogether, the outcome was the same. Many ASC partners and family members displayed a lack of realisation that their self-protective behaviours were also influencing factors to the issues that the resulting problems produced in the relationship. Frequently, their mind-blindness (Baron-Cohen, 1997) appeared to contribute to a belief that their partner and/or family members caused these problems. Rather than recognise their own lack of communicative ability and resulting need to withdraw from communication, those with ASC seemed to perceive that they were often liable for incidents of which they were entirely unaware, therefore innocent. Jim illustrated his unwitting need to avoid communicating because he 'gets disappointed in her behaviour' therefore, obviously he was innocent, and she needed to 'get over it'. However, in the process, he completely missed that she was prompting him to help him to 'try better' to interact with her:

She might see something that she is real fired up about, and I'm thinking 'Oh shit. Can't do anything about it, so forget about it', you know ... So as I said I just walk away. I don't bother. Why, why hassle? I have got enough hassle in my life now without adding more. Yeah, I just get disappointed in her behaviour, but get over it. Got to. Well, that's all you can do, but the point is, okay it has happened get over it. The old saying, it's happened you can't do anything about it. Let's get over it and walk away. Build a bridge ... She said, 'well you should try' and I'm thinking, but try at what? You know, and this is where the crux is. She said, 'Well you should be doing something better.' Yeah, but at what? And I'm thinking well okay fine I don't argue, I don't muck around and just keep on plugging ... but for me when someone says you should try more. Yeah, well try at what? It's a big question mark.

William confirmed this interpretation is quite widespread:

And that's this anger problem that we can't understand. And I've read a lot of entries from people writing on the internet forums. It's one of the topics that we cannot understand, these reactions which we were being quiet, all we can do is to be quite neutral, and even that causes anger. What can you do? You can't do anything.

Then he reported how his need to withdraw from communication was involuntary for him:

And in a marriage, you have, the triggers are hit all that more often, so you're always in pain of some sort. So, it's not just a choice of how to act or how to think, how to react, it's involuntary. And overcoming that is, if you can, is part of the question.

William then added how his need to keep himself under 'tight control' was his response to an inability to respond. This may be seen by those who are NT as withdrawing as well:

And of course, it's a spontaneous thing, and what probably makes normal NT behaviour what it is. Respond instantly to emotional responses. Create them from recognising in others. I can't do that so at least I can keep on an even keel by controlling, keeping a tight control. Otherwise, you're going up and down without knowing why.

Andrew displayed an unawareness of a different sort. When asked to describe some positive aspects about his relationship, Andrew could not find anything to say. Instead, he redirected the question by looking inward, gauging his relationship success by his personal financial failure. However, he saw his failure by means of his partner, as if she was his mirror, and not through his own self-awareness:

> It's almost like being with Hazel has made me realise my failures ... most people at our age obviously totally cashed up and I know it's all physical things and outward things, but I always think that is a sort of outwardly show of something that you were inside of you that you got done, that you were successful. I don't know if there's been any positive things come out of it for me. It's just made me realise things about myself. I mean I don't know what Hazel would say, it's a hard one, that ... I know you are looking for a positive, for me to think of something positive and I can't. I just look at myself as ... it has shown me up for what I am.

Then he added how living in a world where 'social' was the standard gave rise to feelings of inadequacy for him. He said that he did not know how to communicate effectively, portraying himself as an 'alien' while at the same time labelling all others that he was trying to communicate with as 'them'. Consequently, handling communication was foreign to him. All the same, he revealed that he was aware that something was missing:

> Well maybe I'm colour-blind in social things ... It's like being put into an alien world and everyone speaking a different language, so you can't even interface with them ... it is like ... I'm speaking Greek and you are speaking

*Russian and I am going 'I can't communicate there.' That's
a hard one.*

Malcolm's point hit the nail on the head:

*Humans are very emotional. Aspies aren't. Yes. To find a
way in the middle of that is chaotic.*

The Cycle Burdens

The high levels of responsibility that developed within
the prompting practices of NT participants, not only in terms
of relational communication, but also in giving specialised
caring, in being liable for the greater part of family life tasks,
and in handling resulting conflict, resulted in an asymmetrical
development of the relationship. A parental/caretaker role
formed for most NT participants. While most participants
with ASC did not discuss these aspects, Wally did have some
thoughts that he shared on the matter:

*When I get into that state, I need support from her which
she may not be willing to give, and she shouldn't have to
… It puts her into that caring role rather than an equal role
and that's unfair. It's me imposing that need on her that she
shouldn't have to deal with, and it's become a real barrier.
Interesting talking about this stuff because that's what it is,
it's that fear of being the needy one.*

Most NT participants reported that the result of interaction
difficulties and following conflict, for them, was to feel
responsible for assuming a dominant caretaker role while
managing their relationship, which many described as

resembling that of a parent/child relationship. Robyn had earlier written her thoughts about the issue during a course she had previously attended. She read it aloud within the interview:

> *And I, I wrote 'He feels like a child, and I am the parent. He can't cope without me. I have to praise him. I have to prompt him. I have to guide him. I have to teach him. I feel heavy and overburdened. No wonder so many AS-NT couples stop having sex. I just want him to be self-motivated.'*

Then she added how her relationship suffered in the times when she withheld the extra effort:

> *Oh, we don't want to be near each other or with each other if we are both in that state, because an AS person needs a lot of positive feedback, which is a parenting role and doesn't seem to have any inner resources to build themselves up. They need to have someone outside telling them how wonderful they are, which is probably why they make good employees. If they do their job well, and they get good feedback they probably prefer to be at work than at home … but when I am too busy to give positive feedback, our relationship tends to fall over and disintegrate into shouting matches.*

She went on to say that Phil, her husband with ASC, struggled with this aspect as well:

> *So, from his perspective he wants someone to show him 'How do you stay positive when there are so many things you can't remember in a day, and you are always being reminded of what you did wrong?' … Sometimes he gets sick of working so hard all the time. He just wants a simple life and a simple wife. Hahaha.*

The Cycle Ensnares

Like Robyn, many NT participants mentioned impressions of feeling more like a mother or a caretaker, with a continual burden to nurture, look after and manage their partner/family members with ASC:

SABRINA   *It's like having a conversation with a child … If we're not talking business, he's being childlike and I feel like I'm mothering him and I don't want to be that person … He tells me … 'Stop trying to be my mother' and I'm like 'Stop acting like a 15-year-old,' so the conversation is like with a kid.*

QUINN   *When I have conversations with him about our relationship, it feels like a mum and a child … I feel it's like a mum is getting onto the child and then the child is trying to do something to kind of calm mum down … but it's also, how teenagers think they know everything, and you know nothing, and that's where you go, you have not got beyond being a 15-year-old boy. I hear my son kind of behaves like that … I say to him 'You think you know everything', but you can't be a wife and a mother and be married to someone who behaves and treats you as though you're 15 and you're in a 15-year-old relationship.*

DEREK   *In many ways I suppose I've … given up on trying to have any more of an instructive role because to me it feels that I'm just being like a teacher and a carer and not being a partner … I find that, at times [it] can get frustrating, asking for a level of detail that is really onerous.*

DIANNE   *You are the fixer, you are the direction giver, you're the one who has to take charge again, and feel like a mother, or a carer, or a do this, do that, like with your kids you know … So yeah, it is just frustrating. You are taking charge again. You are having to make decisions again. You having to take on the burden again and it's that sharing thing that doesn't happen. It is not, 'Let's do this together, what do you think?' 'Cause, they don't have an opinion. It is like, 'Well I don't know, so you tell me.' Yeah, it's just annoying … I could be more responsive, and I could go, 'What a great job. That's fantastic', but I feel like I am talking to a 10-year-old child and I'm just, you know … Naaa. And hey, if you can do that, that's great but I'm just past it … Provided he is given a direction to take, its fine, but left to deal with it on his own, and make those decisions, and to know, 'What should I do about this', yeah, not good. But with, 'well okay let's do this', and 'let's do that', and 'how about you do this', and he is given direction, he will be up on a higher scale. But on his own. No.*

When asked how she felt, she replied:

Fairly annoyed because I feel like a mother leaving a list for the kids to do, or for, the person to come in, because if you don't leave a list then it doesn't get done. There is nothing, like, the thought is not like, 'Dianne is at work so what I could do today is vacuum, or I could clean the bathroom or … '. If I leave a list and go, 'can you do these things' it will be done, but not done spontaneously. And as I mentioned before with lists around things about when you have sex or when you do this yeah that really pisses me off. I just think, no I would rather just go without, it is all too hard. If I live my life by lists around those things that I feel just should happen in a relationship, well that would drive me crazy. But when there are jobs … that's how he gets his own self-esteem. He does a job, and he finishes it. The only thing is if I write a list and he achieves the whole list and I don't go, 'Wow that's great', then, 'I did everything on the list', so you feel like his mother or his teacher. I sometimes get a bit sarcastic and sometimes say, 'Well I didn't bring the gold stars home today, but I will get them tomorrow.'

LUCY   *I guess it's almost like training a child … You don't expect to be doing that when they're in their fifties and sixties … I believe that yes, I am the major caretaker … being the caretaker of the emotional side … but I seem to be the one working at it all the time … You've just got to point it out to him. He just doesn't get it because he's so focused on him. I guess that's the childlike way that they go about things … It's not that they have no emotion in my opinion, it's just that it's so childish. Very, very childlike … unless we're talking about his stuff, it's as if they're of little interest to him.*

RONDA

I feel resentment ... because having to mother that person all these years detracted from the mothering that I owed my children and when I think back now on all those countless, countless evenings at the supper table ... when he and I would just be sitting at the table arguing, arguing, arguing, arguing. Never going anywhere. Never getting any resolution. Just going round in these ridiculous crazy circles all evening long ... It detracted from the quality of mothering that I owed my children ... because my children, all six children greatly, greatly suffered because of this relationship between this Asperger person and myself.

KAY

So I am constantly telling him things. I feel like his mother. He gets insulted [be]cause his mum passed when he was about eight or nine, so now I change it to 'I feel like the adult, and you are the child.' He gets insulted and he says, 'No it is not that way at all.' Yes, it is actually.

DIANA

I have to prompt him and try to explain to him that I'm not trying to mother him, I'm not trying to be like his mother.

RYAN

Yeah, look if there is peace to be made, I am mostly the person that makes the peace and so if there is an apology to be given, even if it is not my fault, I will apologise just to keep things on an even keel and some of that was explained to Rachelle to how other relationships work.

Some NT participants also commented that they struggled with the decision to stay in the relationship and continue with the resulting exhaustion and health issues that living in an almost constant state of conflict caused. However, some revealed an accompanying guilt with the desire to leave. Some also expressed concern that their partner/family members with ASC would not be able to cope alone. Fiona said as much:

But I really don't see the solution. At this stage in my life, splitting up, we've been together too long. I just feel if I walked away from it that he would be this lost person. He would be by himself with no connection with the outside world, and it's not, it's not pity that I feel for staying with him, it's just compassion. One human being to another.

In Summary

In neurodiverse relationships, the alternating struggle between individual needs, and striving to get individual needs met, results in incompatible behaviours of prompting and self-protection between ASC and NT adults. These incompatible behaviours are both the main contributing factor in the formation of the prompt dependency cycle, and also the main contributing factors in the continuation of the prompt dependency cycle. Neither ASC or NT participants were able to overcome both, their diametrically opposed needs, and their widely divergent behaviours, which was a result of striving for these opposing needs. There is clear evidence that the most satisfied people within close relationships are those who do not avoid communication about important relational topics, or conflicts, and instead develop a sense of working together through their difficulties (Gottman & Notarius, 2002). However, the incompatible needs of each, and the resulting alternating struggle seemed to counteract any chance of those within neurodiverse relationships to be able adopt collaborative practices with each other. A sense of working together was unable to develop in the majority of neurodiverse relationships, with very little option for either person to do anything differently.

The main effect of the prompt dependency cycle on both ASC and NT participants was to become entwined in a power struggle that, in turn, formulated a parental/caretaker role for NT participants. This role positioned NT participants with the obligation of managing their relationship, taking care of their partner/family members and being responsible for holding their relationship together. Rather than being able to enjoy the rapport, attachment and connection expected within close relationships, most of the NT participants (both male and female), relayed the notion that they did not really have a relationship at all; that they had no-one to rely on or help them when they needed support, which created a sense of 'aloneness' in the relationship for them. A variety of negative feelings such as frustration, anger and loneliness developed for them.

Thus, the interlocked, constant and unresolvable circular conversations and communication difficulties accompanied by the avoidant and self-protective behaviours on the part of ASC, and prompting behaviours on the part of NT, emerged as natural by-products of the ongoing endeavours, by each, to get needs met. The resulting high levels of burden for NT participants and the ongoing communication roundabout with its entangled communication and subsequent friction, was found to give rise to the formation of additional communication cycles throughout the prompt dependency cycle. We look at these additional interconnected communication cycles and the subsequent effect on each in the next chapter.

9

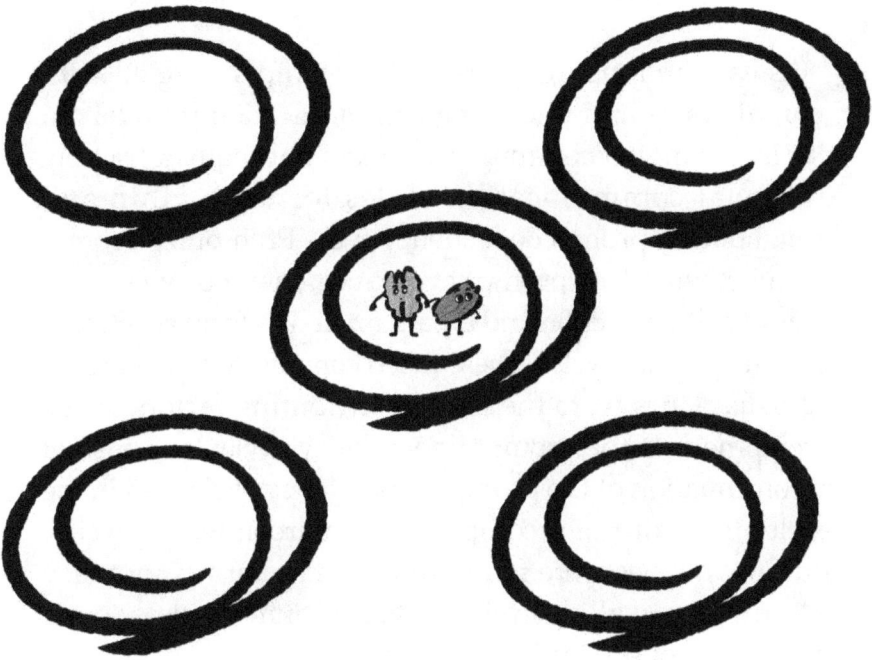

The Cycle Multiplies

'The art of conversation is the art of hearing as
well as being heard.'
William Hazlitt

Caught in a Trap

As each in a neurodiverse relationship struggled with
the unalterable and unceasing communication roundabout
with its entangled communication and subsequent friction,
additional communication cycles formed within and
throughout the prompt dependency cycle. Prompting, prompt
dependency and/or prompt avoidance, merged with other
forms of self-protection and amalgamated to form additional
communicational cycles. These fused complicated interactions
and behaviours were the main contributing factors in the
development of the prompt dependency cycle, the cause of
the continuation of the prompt dependency cycle, and in the
development of the accompanying interconnected cycles.
Additional cycles were found to be the imitating normalcy
cycle, the stonewalling cycle, the help seeking cycle, and the
loss of sense of self cycle.

Imitating Normal

Normalcy is a social construct that is defined through
culture, media, and the standard codes of conduct and rules
of communities (Lasser & Corley, 2008). Since adults with
ASC often appear similar to NT adults, the compensation
strategies and coping mechanisms they use can conceal their
difficulties in public (Rench, 2014). Decisions about disclosure

are accompanied by the fear of stigma and bias. Lingsom (2008) suggests that although this decision is about protecting personal privacy, when trying to pass as 'normal', those with invisible impairments are constructing multiple and conflicting identities that challenge conventional categories, thereby promoting a narrow view of normality. Lingsom (2008) adds that this hiding of reality contributes nothing to dismantling social and structural barriers to participation, belonging and wellbeing of all people. Even so, keeping a socially accepted façade was a construct that both ASC and NT participants endeavoured to uphold, and in public both ASC and NT participants tried to appear 'normal'. The normalcy cycle involves the disconnect between what occurs in the privacy of the home and what occurs in public. This cycle informed and intertwined with many aspects of the prompting and self-protective cycles, given that NT participants reported that they often fill in the missing gaps of standard social information for their partner/family members with ASC. Murray (ASC) shared that his partner had helped him to learn social rules:

Over time I've picked up a lot of rules ... when Jane has explained to me 'You shouldn't say this or you should do it that way or whatever' because I've come from being fully clueless to being, I now know a lot of them intellectually ... I think for people who are on the spectrum that don't have partners that explain the rules to them they would know less of the rules ... every social rule needs to be explained ... if my partner never explained the rules to me, I literally wouldn't know them.

In interviews, ASC participants revealed that they were aware of the usual social conventions but unaware of generally accepted social conventions for the maintenance of close relationships. They discussed the differences between how they functioned at home and at work and their views about the differences between their public and private lives:

> RICHARD   *The actual day in, day out, married life ... and what's normal ... you're pretty much learning things as you go along ... When you go out the front door ... you put on a happy face, and you say 'Good day' to everybody but ... at home it could be World War Three ... but you don't take that outside.*

> BARRY   *We have sort of parallel lives where she is doing her thing and I am doing my thing ... I suppose Aspies are comfortable with that unless something goes wrong ... I suppose from someone who is looking on the outside in, they would say 'Oh it's not the most ... affectionate goings-on'.*

While those with ASC can benefit from the support given to them by their partner/family members to help them navigate the nuances of affection and connection and also construct normalcy in their lives, NT participants reported that it was a different story for them. Given that reading body language is a common difficulty for those on the spectrum, NT participants described the ways in which they had to adapt to a different way of approaching affection, connection and relating, behind closed doors, while also facing a disconnect in public. They shared that this difference between the public persona, and the person that they experienced behind closed doors created a gulf between the actual and the artificially constructed aspects of their lives:

KATY   *I mean, it's a weird feeling to sit and be
            absolutely distraught and crying and have him
            change the subject and say, 'I saw the most
            amazing engine the other day.' You are in
            the middle of this terrible crisis and breaking
            your heart, and he is telling you about nuts
            and bolts. I mean, that defies all reasoning.
            So, you don't talk to people about that.*

TRACY   *At first, I did not dare to tell anyone ... then,
            after seeking professional help, I felt more
            at ease about sharing with more people ...
            because James is a totally different person in
            public.*

DIANA   *I suppose for my husband, subtle things you
            can do just kind of go straight over his head,
            and there is a bit of lack of, I suppose of caring
            for even the needs or wants of somebody else.
            It does seem that he's quite self-centred a
            lot of the time but I'm sure he doesn't really
            mean to be. He's really got quite a nice nature
            underneath it all, but sometimes I suppose
            you can take it personally, because it comes
            across kind of a bit callous or insensitive but
            yeah, he doesn't mean to be.*

MANDY   *We went and got diagnosed, so he understands
            it as well now so we can talk about it ... that
            I'm able to express to him the frustration and
            why, and it's not having a go at him as much.
            It's just explaining that that's normal for him.
            I just have to learn to live with it ... I said to*

him 'Don't tell your mum that we've had it diagnosed', but he did ... and she'll say 'You know he doesn't really have Asperger's. He's not on the spectrum. He doesn't have any sort of autism.' And I'll say 'Okay, alright', because there's no point, there's no point, but he knows now. So, it's something we can say 'Okay well this is part of why you do it like this, and this is why I do it like this', and we just need to find a common way of solving this problem which usually is me compromising more than anything. But it's a way of being able to, at least I feel like I've discussed it. Whether I've got an answer, or solution, I've still discussed it, so it's off my chest a bit more.

Resisting Normal

Stonewalling is an avoidance tactic used to terminate a conversation (Gottman, 1993; Gottman & Gottman, 2017). Avoiding conversations, becoming defensive to stop a conversation, shutting down to end a conversation, and becoming verbally aggressive to stop a conversation, can all be termed stonewalling behaviour. Stonewalling was a recurring behaviour displayed regularly by ASC participants and often presented as a sort of abrasiveness that overlooked the perspective of others. The stonewalling cycle, brought on by the difficulties and differences with interactions those with ASC experience led to substantial relational problems. Although both ASC and NT participants discussed many occurrences of stonewalling behaviour, many ASC participants did not appear to be that concerned about it:

The Cycle Multiplies

RACHELLE *I don't want the conversation to occur ... Sometimes I tell him I don't understand why it is so much of a big issue ... He does [explain] but I still don't really get it.*

TERRY *When we have some sort of misunderstanding or argument or disagreement I tend to withdraw completely and let things settle down, which I find ... works for me, but it doesn't work for Kim.*

While most NT participants reported an understanding that avoidance of their conversations was not always deliberate, they also reported that the stonewalling behaviour shown to them, and the resulting disconnection, was an extensive challenge to their relationship:

LAURA *He either evades or gets frightened and retreats ... His tendency [is] to get out of uncomfortable things with small lies ... obsessive secrecy, which has grown more as we've been together ... he just blanks me on certain topics.*

RUTH *He would prefer to not talk through issues, which I find odd ... A willingness to talk through issues and listen to the other person is important in a relationship ... Him getting defensive and shutting down, freezing, not answering questions, not talking to me, stonewalling. Sometimes he even walks away from me when I'm talking. He often forgets what we talk about.*

GEORGIA   *They pick up on, they learn what is appropriate,
and what is not appropriate in certain social
situations. I think that if they'd lived with a
person for long enough, they learn how to
manipulate them, and they'll use that skill
to their advantage, and I think that that is
intentional. It's almost like a Jekyll and Hyde
… you can see they have the potential to be
kind and they're not always … but then they
can flip and that's when the other side, it's
almost like the other side of their brain is
well, 'I need this right now so I'm going to do
whatever it takes to have my needs fulfilled
and if that means making that person back
down these are the things that I'm going to
say to that person'. That's intentional!*

Then Georgia added that she had read a book about the life
of a man on the spectrum. She commented on the difference
of the attitude of the person in the book as compared to her
husband and what it meant for their relationship:

*I just thought wow what a difference in opinion, you've got
one person saying, 'Well if we'd have known we could have
done something about it' and then we've got another one who
is saying 'Well if we'd have known I still wouldn't have done
… anything about it', because I was stronger more belligerent,
more cocky, more confident, more set in … you know it's my
way or the highway type of thinking and I thought that was
interesting … When it's undiagnosed and you go through a
bunch of shit and you get hurt trying … and then you get the
diagnosis, trying to put the hurt … and it's on both sides, I
mean I know I have to … take responsibility for me hurting*

182

him too … It must be hard for someone with Asperger's to have this woman raging at you, because sometimes you have to rage at them because you're like so fricking frustrated! … 'Why are you … ?' He goes 'Well why are you so angry?' And I'm not angry. I'm so frustrated. There's a difference, anger no, frustration yes! … And you can't even have any intonation in your voice! How can you just be, if you can't be your emotional self? … I've said to people I would have to speak, you know how counsellors speak in that voice where they talk to you … I'm like, ha that doesn't come naturally to me, when I'm dealing with a relationship, a close intimate relationship where there's emotions involved.

Seeking Normal

Seeking help was found to be a complicated issue for most participants. The seeking help cycle was the cause of much heartache. The invisible nature of adults on the autism spectrum, together with the effort involved in keeping a socially accepted façade, resulted in both ASC and NT participants facing either disbelief or rejection when seeking help.

Most of those with ASC said that they did not seek help or talk to family and friends about their relationships. Those who did seek help, either through family and friends or professionally, reported varying degrees of success. When asked if he talked to friends and family about his relationship Terry said:

No. I've never done that, the only person I discuss my relationship with is Kim.

The he added that he had sought professional help, which was not always positive:

> We've been through a number of psychologists ... I went to one psychiatrist who just didn't believe it ... I referred to some of the other people that I'd seen which included Tony Attwood, and just about any adult with a diagnosis of Asperger's pretty well knows who Tony Attwood is ... and he'd never heard of him so he sort of wasn't sure about this diagnosis ... I think I only saw him two or three times and decided, no that wasn't going to work for me because I think he thought that I was not on the spectrum.

Similarly, Murray explained that he did not talk to others about his relationship:

> No, only because the best person to talk to is my wife and ... I don't feel like I need to talk to others ... I think naturally Asperger people aren't that keen to talk about their emotions.

Likewise, Daniel said that he did not talk to family or friends either:

> No. Apart from Cathy I don't really have friends, and my family adds up to two grown sons and a father; autistic too, I believe, who's pushing ninety and profoundly deaf.

He added:

> Early on, there was a time when Cathy despaired of my social ineptitude and overall weirdness. Then the autism diagnosis came along, and there isn't anyone who knows any more

The Cycle Multiplies

than we do about that. We sought any available help early on. Now we don't bother.

When asked about seeking help, Barry said:

I wouldn't be able to pinpoint what, if someone said, 'Okay now what's the problem?' You ... managed to find a counsellor say, and then I don't know how to answer that, I would go 'Uh, ah, yeah, good question, ah I don't know.' A lot of the time ... you can't put your finger on what you think is wrong ... when I think of it in hindsight, compared to what other people go through, I think Hope and I have had ... a pretty good relationship.

However, William outlined his rejection of help:

Nah, I deal with it myself. Don't need it. I tried it a couple of times and it winds up being an intellectual challenge between me and the counsellor, and I always win, in my opinion ... all the talking and counselling in the world, which is what Fiona is inclined to go along with, at the end of the day, it is my decision as to how I deal with things, what I listen to, and what I do and if there is any changes to be made I need to do it. And I think it is whether I want to change.

On the other hand, Samuel said that he did talk to one friend, and he had sought out professional help as well:

Yeah, my friend at work that I sit next to ... has been through very similar relationship experiences to me and at least we're able to sit and talk frankly to each other and that does help, yeah ... Someone who doesn't judge you and just lets you talk. Oh yes, we went to Eleanor Giddens for a while ...

Have They Gone Nuts?

Eleanor was great. But she is a specific practitioner in adult Asperger's, so I imagine she's heard it all … It certainly gave us some handy tips, but at the end of the day, if we didn't want to do it … again it's led us to this situation.

Sandra said that she had talked with a therapist, but talking with family and friends was a different story:

When it comes to talking to friends and family, it doesn't really occur to me to talk to them about that stuff you know whether it's my husband or my kids … it just doesn't occur to me to talk to them about my personal life, unless it's going to affect them … When I started seeing a therapist after a few years, I think it kind of helped just talking stuff out, you know but then I think after a while I kind of get back into kind of the way things were again because that's what ends up kind of coming natural again.

Rachelle shared the long journey that led to her diagnosis:

I saw … in the twenties, psychologists and psychiatrists and doctors and counsellors etc. etc., trying to work out what was wrong and then finally my son was diagnosed and then I was diagnosed … now I know, everything came together as one, like I finally, it finally has a label.

However, Mareena said that she had become the counsellor:

Well, I do the talking bit … I've had a lot of counselling and psychotherapy and stuff like that and now I'm counselling other people and I'm managing our office and all those things, I feel that I'm as competent as anyone else and probably I have discovered some counsellors are actually not necessarily

on my wavelength and also if they are not themselves on the
spectrum, they will not be helpful.

When NT interviewees were asked about seeking help, most reported that talking with others was a delicate issue. Many reported that inadequate community knowledge and limited awareness about adults on the spectrum, led to them feeling invisible and disbelieved. While they made it clear that they would welcome being able to talk through their difficulties with others, the lack of understanding and resulting opinions and conclusions that others arrived at resulted in mixed reactions. For this reason, many had selected the 'not applicable' option in their survey to the two statements about being believed by family, friends and professionals. Seeking professional help was also reported to cause mixed results. Sophie reported on the difficulties that she met from the lack of community understanding:

> *I usually do not [talk about it] because others have no concept*
> *of what I go through or deal with. The issues ... of an AS*
> *man does not resemble anything from a normal NT – NT*
> *relationship for people to relate to. The few times I do reach*
> *out ... their response quickly reminds me I shouldn't have*
> *reached out to them ... Unless someone has gone through a*
> *relationship like ours, there is no way for them to relate to*
> *this experience ... I find some friends incredibly judgemental*
> *of him, and us, so I retreat further away from them.*

Wanda gave details of the difficulties of explaining the distinct problems to others:

> *I find when you talk to friends ... or colleagues it's more*
> *'Oh all men are like that' ... You don't really feel that you're*

listened to or understood … Other people see your spouse …
his talent and he's able to communicate in a very professional
manner to other people … and you're like, you don't live
with it … Always not believed!

Whereas Laura mentioned that a partner's arrogance can
stop the potential to get help:

He wouldn't participate. Contemptuous of psychiatry, and
what is there to work on, anyway!

Sabrina was fortunate to have understanding friends:

Luckily, I've got friends that have been around him, so they
know that he's a little different, so I don't deal with the
disbelief that I think some people have encountered.

Losing Normal

A common result of the unresolvable communication
differences and resultant consequences for both NT and ASC
participants was a sense of a loss of self. This cycle was the
cause of much heartache. Felt by both groups of participants,
a loss of self was experienced for very different reasons. Many
of the participants with ASC mentioned the necessity to fit
into the neurotypical world, and what that meant to them in
their day-to-day lives:

DANIEL   *For the first half century of my life, I had*
a sense of purpose – making sense of the
world. Then … I discovered autism. Another
decade or so of research and I'm left high and

dry – there's no place in the world for adult autistics. We're there, but we conspire to maintain our ignorance. A bit like climate change really, which is likely to take us all out long before our socialised autistic children have had time to change the world.

Most NT participants mentioned that their sense of self became lost as they often had to capitulate to the continual rigidity of their partner/family members with ASC. They felt grief over the loss of the person they once were:

QUINN   *I no longer know who I am. I think that's probably the most painful part of this whole thing ... I've lost myself ... I love him but I want to get myself back ... I was very outgoing and a 'happy-go-lucky' kind of girl and I always liked to help people and I felt like I was happy and full in my life and that's not the way I feel anymore ... I have no idea who I am anymore.*

RYAN   *When you are inside the family unit, I feel very much that it is team Rachelle and not team [us] so ... yeah, I do feel like it's the loss of myself, in a lot of ways ... It is really very much about what she wants, and wants to do, and wants to achieve, and not really much about what I want ... I'm very quick to make a sacrifice ... for the rest of my family ... I'm trying to manage a relationship that all works ... Yes thinking about others.*

RENEE   *That's a real big focus for me, is to work out who I am, or who I was and who I am now ... because you live with someone else's reality and I find myself more and more challenging his view of reality because for so many years I thought that ... his view of reality, that was the right one.*

GEORGIA   *I was a go-getter. I had drive and I had energy and determination ... but coming out of this relationship it's like I've lost that sense of self-esteem ... If you're told enough that you're a bird brain, and you don't understand, and that you're wrong, and your view of the world is wrong, and you don't understand how people in the world work and that you're stupid, you start believing it ... You start losing sense of self, and you feel just an extension of them and if you assert yourself and your own opinions and your own needs then ... my own experience has been that it's put down or told that you're wrong or told that you don't live in the real world ... and you're totally invalidated and so then you start the second guessing, well I shouldn't be feeling like this because he's told me I shouldn't be feeling like this, this is not the way to respond ... You don't want to become the yes person, you end up becoming the yes person, because their ability to convince you that your way is wrong or the way you're thinking is wrong because you don't agree with the way they're thinking, just breaks you down.*

The Cycle Multiplies

LILLY   *I went to see Carers Victoria at one stage ... and got some support for me ... and the lady who I saw... said 'So ... what does Lilly want?' And I go 'I'm stuck. I'm absolutely speechless.' I had no idea. Still sort of don't, ha, ha. However, I understand that I have lost the sense of myself ... I still know that I have needs and desires and stuff like that, but you put your own self on the backburner to try to find the best possible way to enrich their lives. However, I am going to flip that again because I believe what I am learning is, I've just got to keep building myself up, to be a person and do what I love.*

RONDA   *We learn about ourselves by the reactions other people have to us. That's just how we learn about ourselves and then we adjust. Now the fact that he has Asperger's, now I understand this, but for years it was so confusing it was just so confusing, you know it was like the frog being slowly boiled in the pot. You don't realise that you're losing your sense of self until all of a sudden one day you're really depressed or you're really confused or really anxious ... In hindsight now that I know about Asperger's, I realise ... but over the years I've felt this you know being reflected back to me was 'You're a threatening person, you're a scary person' and so I would try to adapt in my ignorance. I would try to adapt and be less scary, less threatening, more subdued, more-soft spoken, more cooperative, more consolatory, more, more, more. Of course, it never worked.*

In Summary

The constant interplay between prompting on the part of NT adults and self-protective and/or dependency behaviours on the part of ASC adults were the basis of the development of the prompt dependency cycle. The evolution of this communication cycle into a dynamic communication system with additional interconnected cycles was the result of the endless cycles of unsolvable communication imbedded in the prompt dependency cycle. The imitating normalcy cycle, the stonewalling cycle, the help seeking cycle, and the loss of sense of self cycle arose from the challenges of incapacities of each to negotiate and reconcile a deprivation of needs for affection and connection on the part of adults who are NT, and solitude on the part of adults with ASC.

A further consequence of the dynamic communication system that formed within neurodiverse relationships was unresolved disappointment, anxiety, depression and anger for NT individuals. Not only did NT participants have to endure misinterpretations of their intentions from their ASC partner/family members, but they also had to contend with incorrect assumptions from others, such as friends, family and professionals. The invisible nature of adults on the autism spectrum, together with the effort involved in keeping a socially accepted façade, not only caused both groups of people to face disbelief and/ or rejection when seeking help, but also when just wanting to speak with others. A condition known as the Cassandra Phenomenon can sometimes result from this disbelief. The Cassandra Phenomenon is a condition of depression or ill-health that develops from the isolation and loneliness of knowing a truth, experiencing that truth, but not being believed. These issues are discussed in the next chapter.

10

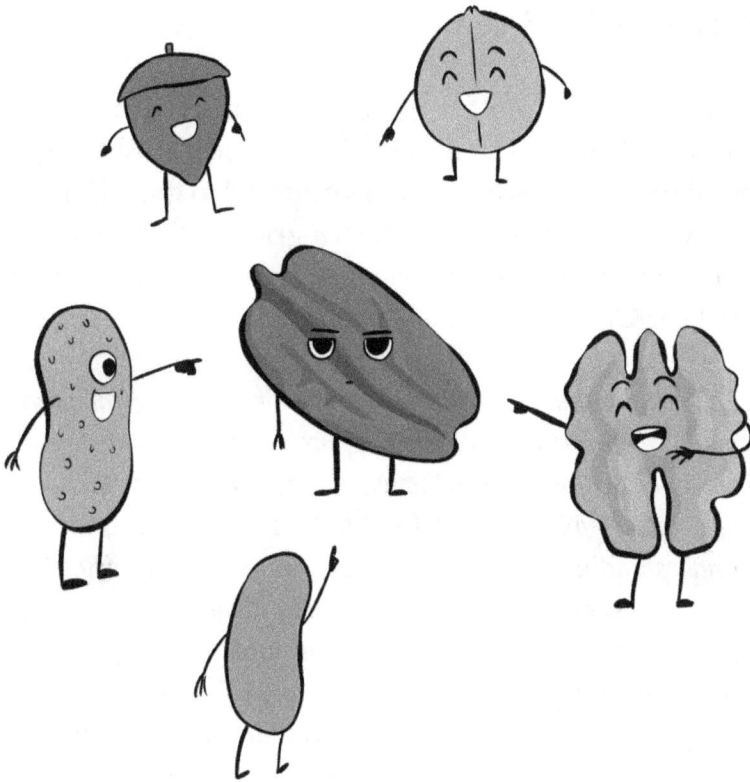

The Arrival of
Cassandra

'All relationships have one law.
Never make the one you love feel alone, especially
when you're there.'
Unknown

Relief, Grief and Unbelief

For some people on the autism spectrum, gaining awareness of autism can come as a relief when attributing past negative experiences to autism as opposed to the self (Hickey et al., 2017). Others can experience grief at the discovery of autism. For others, the knowledge can be quite challenging. Daniel (ASC) described it as 'a curse':

Each communication rubs my nose in deficiency. Any word might be a trapdoor to conflict. Apprehensive is an intelligent reactive posture. For me, knowing about autism is something of a curse, which can't be lifted without an improved understanding of what it is … across the community. I'm part of a generation who will, generally, die without knowing they're different, and that improved understanding might never come to pass. I spend most of my conscious hours in an office. Autism in adults is significant to the organisational dynamics but forms no part of the conversations. As far as I know, I'm the only one who's autistic and knows about it, and I'm instructed to respect the ignorance of the others. I fought recently to have mention of cognitive difference included in the organisation's psychological wellbeing policy, but I'll be retired before that gets beyond draft. I have been trained, along with the rest of the organisation, in interview techniques that encourage discrimination against candidates with inappropriate eye or hand movements. I spent four years as the only autistic on the board of our local support organisation. I know there's nothing to be done for us. I believe very strongly in the need for full grown autistics and people with more normal social contexts to understand what's going on. Apprehension doesn't hold me back; realistic assessment of costs, risks and benefits does.

However, Georgia (NT) conveyed her relief after many years of living in a state of confusion, doubt, and loss:

I thought I should be trying to change myself to make things better. I just blamed myself. I thought I was at fault. I really did! Yeah, your whole reality, or what you believe should be, you keep being told that's not the way it is. So, you have to start trying to think their way, or I'm wrong, or I shouldn't be asking ... always being told that I was demanding too much. If you were crying and you were saying 'I just need your support' or 'Can you just spend an hour with me?' 'Oh, you're just too demanding' or 'you're too sensitive'. That was a common one ... and I would start to believe 'I'm too sensitive, I overreact' and then when you get to counselling and they say, 'No you have feelings, and you feel things.' And then you suppress those feelings ... and it depends what you decide to do with those feelings ... At one point, instead of taking them on, and acknowledging them, and accepting them, and saying 'I can have these feelings. It's okay', I tried to stuff them away and try and say that it's not okay to feel like this. I shouldn't be feeling like this. And ... that was really, really destructive. I became that – I don't know who I am. Two and a half years ago, I would just look in the mirror and just look at myself and go 'Who am I?' And I still do that ... I feel like I've lost just some part of me inside ... I'm trying to get back that, what I call 'the real me', 'the old me'. I'm a different me, or I've become more truly me. I'm allowing myself now to be me, but when we were in the thick of it, it was dark.

Childish Allusions

While a growing awareness of autism in a relationship is a complicated issue, it is particularly problematical in the wider community. Added burden can be placed on people in neurodiverse relationships from incorrect assumptions others (such as friends, family and professionals) can develop due to the invisibleness of adults on the autism spectrum. Accounts by NT participants revealed that the parental/caretaker role that they were required to adopt, played a part in maintaining others' misreading of their words and actions:

DAWN   *He will look at you like you are talking at him like he is an idiot … [I] have to assume that … [he's] not going to share that information with me … When people observe us as a couple, they think I am treating him like a kid at times … I know he thinks like that sometimes, but if I don't ask, I will never know, I won't get told, because I know it doesn't cross his mind to tell me or he thinks he has told me.*

RUTH   *We went to regular marriage counselling with a pastor. He addressed some of the issues; a lot was related to communication issues but didn't understand the root of the issues or seem to get that my husband lacked common sense, empathy, and the ability to see my*

perspective on anything. He did seem to get
that my husband was immature and focused
on himself. He made comments like 'I'm
pretty sure he can handle that' in reference to
some parenting things and dressing the kids
appropriately for the weather, etc., and I just
shook my head 'No!'

Notions of Irrationality

All NT participants interviewed, repeatedly mentioned how difficult it was to live within the consequences of the prompt dependency cycle, its complex system of circular conversations, and its resultant 'caretaker' obligations. It was the stability of the different positions of each group of participants toward interaction and emotional connectedness that was found to equally forefront the durability of the cycling communication and also how it became interwoven within most aspects of communication within these relationships. Most interviewed, recognised that a considerable part of the issues resulted from the communicational difficultly and differences in which constant prompting was a central theme, however their inability to solve the number of continuing problems led many to question their own sanity. Dianne shared her struggles with the unrelenting 'roundabout' revealing that at times she felt as if she was 'losing it':

It is quite stressful. It can get quite stressful, and again
initially in our relationship it was something that I just did,
but it did add to the stress, and you probably didn't realise it.
I think these days it just makes me really resentful, which is
a type of anger, I guess ... I get angry with myself that I still

do it. It is almost like if I don't, I feel guilty because then he is left on his own ... and 'gee what happens if', you know, so you feel guilty if you don't, and so it creates a resentment and then I get angry with myself, because I think 'Well why are you still doing this? You don't need to do this. This is just bullshit, you know, you are still doing it', but you feel guilty if you don't. So, I probably, it just makes me think 'oh my God here we go again', so you're on that roundabout round and round ... Over the years there has probably been lots of tears shed. I would go away and cry a lot. I don't know. I actually have over the years probably thought there are times when I probably had mini breakdowns about like, 'oh my god, I'm just falling apart, like physically falling apart'. Just go 'I can't do this anymore'. And then there are times when you think you are going nuts. You think you're the one totally losing it.

Katy described the exhaustion involved in being entangled in the cycle:

I find it exhausting. I find it absolutely exhausting that we can't have a normal interactive communication ... it's an impossible thing to do. And I guess in a way I've moved further and further towards having that kind of interaction with other people. I don't even imagine that I am going to be able to have it with him.

When asked how she felt about the situation, she replied:

At the time? I feel devalued. I feel assaulted verbally. I guess in a way I feel diminished and on the whole very frustrated. Intensely frustrated that it is the same old, same old, and he will actually feedback the information that I am saying the same things. And when I say to him, 'Well it's the same issues come up over and over again and then not resolved' … I may say the same things, but they are unresolved. That becomes very frustrating.

Like Dianne, Katy also pointed to the impact that the communication issues had on her mental health:

I went through that period where I questioned my own sanity. I thought well 'is that what I said?' Because he can actually twist my words to something so unpleasant, that it is completely contrary to the kind of person I am, and then I begin questioning whether I actually did say it like that, or I did say something, so I mean when you think about all this, they're almost impossible to live with, really.

Robyn discussed mental health issues as well:

You just have to be a woman and go to one of those support groups or Katrin's seminars to know that these women, if they are not mentally unhinged, they are very close to it … everyone tried to give the synopsis briefly, but most people failed because once they start talking, they're just an emotional mess … Is it possible to keep your mental health and have a long-term relationship with an Aspie?

When asked how she felt about this issue, she stated:

Tired. Worn out. Bitter. Depressed. Lose hope. Not interested in physical intimacy.

Kay described how lonely her relationship had become because of the never-ending cycle. She revealed that she dealt with the situation by initiating some of the distance herself:

> *I am angry and disappointed, and I am sad. I feel more isolated. I feel as though I am on my own … and do everything myself … I feel alone. Yeah, I feel as though I carry the weight in the marriage. I feel I am pushed into a position of, I am the one. I am it. Yeah. I am it … I leave him out of the loop. Yeah, I've become a bit more guarded. I leave him out of the loop.*

Not only did NT participants experience intense feelings of self-doubt, but they also often encountered daily and subtle forms of incorrect conclusions from others, their partners and other family members. Other's observations and evaluations of their attempts to make sense of their experiences, led many to question their own sanity. Regularly, others came to similar conclusions:

RUTH
It used to be that I was written off as 'emotional', 'crazy' or my thoughts and feelings about things just didn't make sense to him most of the time. Now, he seems to realise that what I say is valid or important more often than he used to.

RONDA
It's extremely hard because any of the dysfunction they see as coming from me … I was Skyping with my second daughter … but she just threw it back in my face and said 'Oh it's not Asperger's. It's not that at all … He doesn't even have it. It's you that can't get along with anybody' … In families that's why

it's such a tragedy … If you marry someone with Asperger's or you're raised by a parent with Asperger's it absolutely wreaks havoc in a family. Family relationships explode, there's division, there's tension, there's strife, you never have harmonious happy family relationships.

RAE   *If you went into a normal counsellor, I'd … be made the fool, and then they come away more arrogant than ever going 'Well there is nothing wrong with me, it's all you' … Years ago we went and saw the pastors … then he just said to both of them 'Oh Rae does talk a lot.' Well, I will never forget it, the two of them just burst out laughing … 'Rae talks so much … obviously she is just waffling on with gobbledygook' … It's just hard isn't it? No-one really understands.*

WANDA   *I have at different times said … how I'm feeling and … like after two or three days he seems to just react … as if we didn't even have that conversation … everything is back to normal. They forget that you actually were just trying to disclose to them like how really hurt you've been by something … but when it comes to that situation you feel as if you're just the crazy wife that, you'll just get over whatever mood it is you're going through, and everything will be back to normal. I think other women would challenge my sanity, like I haven't made any changes, yeah. But like you say, I don't think they would understand.*

GEORGIA   *If these communication issues are really*
identified and seen that they can have such
devastating effects on couples … I mean just
being validated and knowing … people are
starting to realise it's there, it happens, it's
real and that the suffering … whether you
call it the Cassandra Phenomenon or some
sort of ongoing stress disorder like PTSD …
we do suffer, we suffer as a consequence.

Making Matters Worse

Research has established that the mental health of NT
individuals in neurodiverse relationships are often negatively
affected (Bostock-Ling, 2017; Millar-Powell & Warburton,
2020). For NT individuals, the caregiving role appears to be
one of the main features of being involved in a neurodiverse
relationship, while at the same time, they usually experience
intense struggles in their attempts to resolve a needs deprivation
and connect with their ASC partner/family members. Often
becoming physically and emotionally overwrought in the
process, this battle foreshadows a deterioration in both mental
and physical health. Likewise, feelings of loneliness in their
relationship, due to the limited affection, emotional support
and connection that they receive, often leads to feeling isolated
and alone, due to a lack of belief from outside others.

At times, relational issues in neurodiverse relationships
can lead to physical and psychological abuse (Arad et al.,
2022). A study by Arad et al. (2022) revealed 'that women
in neurodiverse relationships reported being victims of
physical and psychological abuse at a higher rate than

women in neurologically typical relationships' (p. 7). Being on the autism spectrum does not necessarily make a person abusive; however, to avoid challenging communication, behaviour can become controlling or even result in domestic violence (Arad et al., 2022; Aston, 2003; Grigg, 2012). Emotional overreactions caused by difficulties experienced by those on the autism spectrum, either from trying to relate to others, or not wanting to relate, can cause an appearance of ill-intent. Aston (2003) reported that, in her investigations as a psychologist working with Asperger-Neurotypical couples, 40% of men with Asperger's Syndrome indicated that, at some point in their relationship, they had been physically abusive toward their partner, while 70% disclosed that they had been verbally abusive towards their partners. Grigg (2012) states that abuse in its many forms can be a common experience within neurodiverse relationships. Grigg also mentions that the most frequent behavioural descriptions NT people gave of their partners with ASC included 'verbal aggression, blame, disproportionate emotional reactions, frequent criticism, [together with] correction, withdrawal, [and] retaliation' (Grigg, 2012, p. 40). The study conducted by Arad's et al. (2022) supports Grigg's conclusions. Results showed higher rates of 'psychological abuse than physical abuse for women with diagnosed partners and women who suspected their partners to be on the autism spectrum, in comparison with women in neurologically typical relationships' (p. 7).

In these studies, when asked about whether physical ill-treatment had occurred due to conversational frustrations, Diana replied:

You don't really know what's going to trigger him off, so you can feel like you walk around on eggshells but then ... they can sense fear and I can control that so I don't come across fearful … If he doesn't want to do something or doesn't want to cooperate or whatever, he won't, regardless whether it's in a conversation, whether it's something that needs doing, or whatever, and underneath you're sort of often intimidated because you know what he's capable of, and he doesn't mean to be, like he really doesn't mean to be. He feels so ashamed of it afterwards and everything else but that's always underlying.

Such verbal and physical abuse underlies a syndrome known as Post-traumatic Relationship Syndrome (PTRS) (Vandervoort & Rokach, 2003; 2004; 2006), an anxiety disorder that often occurs following physical, sexual or severe emotional abuse in the context of an emotionally intimate relationship. Grigg (2012) states that attempting to find solutions in the context of neurodiverse relationships 'is like living in a constant state of unfinished business, combined with confusion, day in and day out, and is probably quite a significant threat to our mental and emotional health, and our future outlook' (p. 63). Rodman (personal communication, 2010) has suggested that, when the traumatic relationship continues, it should be referred to as Ongoing Traumatic Relationship Syndrome (OTRS) rather than PTRS. Moreover, the resulting unresolved disappointment, anxiety, depression and anger for NT individuals (Aston, 2003; Jacobs, 2006; Marshack, 2009), has the potential to lead to the Cassandra Phenomenon and depression (Rodman, 2003).

Cassandra's Arrival

The Cassandra Phenomenon (CP) is a term describing circumstances in which legitimate warnings or anxieties are scorned or rejected. The term emanates from Greek mythology.[3] Regarding ASC, CP occurs when the partners or family members of adults with ASC seek help, and are not believed by their partners, family members, professionals and community members, resulting in his/her reluctance to report the symptoms (Jennings, 2005; Rodman, 2003). The Cassandra Phenomenon is a condition of depression or ill-health that develops from the isolation and loneliness of knowing a truth, experiencing that truth, but not being believed (Simons & Thompson, 2009). Neurotypical people in neurodiverse relationships worldwide have embraced the Cassandra label, given that the Priestess Cassandra in Greek mythology was given the gift of knowing the truth and the curse of not being believed (Simons & Thompson, 2009). This reality reflects their experience since they realise that their relationships are atypical, but they often find that others, including therapists, are unwilling to accept the truth of their relationships (Simons & Thompson, 2009). This then explains the hidden nature of OTRS, and often results in this aspect of ASC impairments staying invisible (Jennings, 2005). As Rodman (2003) describes when discussing the experience of

---

[3] Cassandra was a daughter of Priam, the King of Troy. Struck by her beauty, Apollo provided her with the gift of prophecy, but when Cassandra refused Apollo's romantic advances, he placed a curse ensuring that nobody would believe her warnings. Cassandra was left with the knowledge of future events but could neither alter these events nor convince others of the validity of her predictions (Aston, 2009; Jacobs, 2006). The Cassandra Phenomenon is also known as Cassandra Affective Disorder (CAD), Cassandra Affective Deprivation Disorder (CADD, Aston, 2003), or Affective Deprivation Disorder (ADD; Simons, 2009) or Post-Traumatic Relationship Syndrome (PTRS; Vandervoort & Rokach, 2004).

people who are NT in neurodiverse relationships, 'we were not believed or listened to by professionals or medical, spiritual, educational or judicial leaders' (p. 23). The lack of validation or invalidation by professionals further worsens the confusion of the partner, resulting in CP and compounding OTRS.

Conversely, Simons and Thompson (2009) report that the terms Cassandra Phenomenon or Cassandra Syndrome have become controversial since those with ASC have mistakenly interpreted it as putting all the 'blame' for all a relationship's dysfunction on the person with ASC, with some viewing the Cassandra terms as reflecting a prejudice against those with ASC. Simons and Thompson (2009) explain that this is not the case, and should in no way be taken to mean that either person in the relationship is actively or deliberately depriving the other or blaming the other. In neurodiverse relationships, the neurological differences create a situation where people are emotionally out of sync with each other and 'it is overly simplistic to say that one partner causes the deprivation of the other. Instead, the reality is that each partner may contribute to the dysfunction in different degrees' (p. 3). Despite this, CP is not so much brought about by the emotional deprivation that is experienced, the phenomenon or syndrome is created by the effect of not being believed about the experience of emotional deprivation. Therefore, the lack of belief and feeling 'unheard' are the actual cause of CP. When recognition and belief in the person's experiences occurs, the symptoms can be relieved, to a certain extent. Rae (NT) shared what she had read:

> *My doctor told me to look up after Isaac had spent an hour with my psychologist, and she said, 'I think you'll find he has got Asperger's' and I said 'What!' Anyway, when I read*

it, I read that it said the hardest part for the spouse of an Aspie is to explain to their family and friends what it is like ... Nobody gets it ... and they wonder, they wonder why I am so angry all the time!

Grigg (2012) suggests that CP is not an experience exclusive to NT individuals. Grigg proposes that those on the spectrum can also experience CP. When they are aware of their difficulties and choose to seek help, the lack of knowledge many professionals exhibit, may cause those with ASC to remain 'unheard, judged or misdiagnosed' and trigger similar feelings to those felt by NT individuals (p. 33). Wally (ASC) described his experience of a lack of belief:

I find people do not believe the extent of the difficulties that I have personally in day-to-day activity and particularly because I function well at work and I've spoken to other people about this, that you know, work is the place where you know your place, you know your structure, you know your boundaries there are limitations to the subjects that are discussed.

Grigg's recommendation is that once a person receives validation and support, gains awareness that different neurologies are the source of difficulties and confusion, and affronts have been identified, the journey toward moving out from under CP's negative influence can begin (Grigg, 2012). However, these matters are not easily accomplished. Many participants discussed the risks involved in talking with others, which was an often complex issue, with no easy answers. The preconceived notions many exhibited, due to their lack of awareness, often lead to tough or awkward conversations that caused much distress:

HOLLY   *I've had one friend who gave me an absolute*
          lambasting. She's, needless to say, no longer
          a friend, but she took me out after about a
          year and said to me 'For goodness' sake, pull
          yourself together. Jack's not the problem.
          You're the problem.' More or less 'you've just
          got to get over it', and every time she'd say,
          'So what's he doing?' and I'd say, 'such and
          such'. 'Oh, my husband does that' and so she
          just totally wrote off everything I said. And
          then she said to me 'Well it doesn't matter
          whether Jack's got something wrong with
          him or not, you've just got to get on with it'
          and she belongs to the pull yourself together
          school of counselling and in the end, I had
          no option. I had nowhere to go with her and
          I just had to say, 'Look I'm really sorry that
          we're having a disagreement about this, but
          it's pointless us continuing this conversation
          because you're not hearing how it is for me'
          and so I've chosen not to see her and that's a
          real sadness because I've lost friends over it.

A lack of awareness of the dynamics involved in neurodiverse relationships was a feature to many of the misperceptions people held, as unawareness shaped assumptions that either the person with ASC in the relationship was a belligerent person who ill-treated others, or else the NT person in the relationship was a stressed-out, overanxious person, or both. As a result, many participants reported that talking with others was the cause of much heartache. Sometimes, they found acceptance. Most times not. Frequently, they decided that it was safer to hold back the truth:

The Arrival of Cassandra

LILLY *I think unless you are in with the like-minded people, like yourself, and my friend ... and couple of other people that are like-minded, neurotypicals in a sense don't know the underlying moment-by-moment stress that you can have.*

MANDY *I sent him to the doctor to talk to them about the fact that that's what I thought, and I had a doctor tell him that Asperger's was a children's disorder.*

DAWN *Very occasionally I have vented to my sister, when I have ... gone beyond insanity, but I try not to, because I know she doesn't like him particularly, and I don't want to influence how they see him, and I understand that's not uncommon ... I talked ... with my aunt, who is a professional therapist, and she got it straight away. She was just like 'Oh yeah!' ... I haven't talked to my family about him, about my beliefs, I haven't talked to his family.*

TRACY *At first, I did not dare to tell anyone because I honestly thought I must be doing something wrong and that with patience, love and time, things would work out. Only when they did not, did I confide in a friend. Then, after seeking professional help, I felt more at ease about sharing with more people ... because James is a totally different person in public. I was cautious enough not to tell any people whom I did not trust enough to inform extensively. I do not think that anyone can have just a bit of knowledge about AS and be able to believe or understand what we go through. A little bit of knowledge would, in my opinion, only lead to remarks such as 'My husband is the same', or 'All men are like that'.*

RENEE   *It was only when I started telling the truth to myself, and then others that I was able to then look at how weird things actually were and how different our relationship was, once I started to do that, but when I talked to friends about our situation you know the old phrase 'Oh well that's just men', you know that sort of thing.*

MAGGIE   *I remember years ago I used to talk to people about my issues with Luke and the response would be 'Yeah but my husband does that'. So hence, I have the problem – not him … I pick and choose who I discuss it with. I had a friend that I was talking to a while ago, but when I say, 'No that won't work', then 'I'm not trying. I don't want help. I'm not trying' … that my negativity was stifling her growth. So, I have to be cautious about who I talk to. Yep, yep, I have the problem. I don't put up boundaries, or I'm not strong enough, or I don't really want help at all and 'Luke is such a lovely guy. I don't see what your problem is.' Me and Luke went to, I think this is scary, we went to couples counselling with a psychologist that was supposed to know about*

AS ... the psychologist actually sided with Luke, so if you get a professional that actually understands AS, then they side with the AS, because the AS has the problem, and I have to work around ... I have to do all the work to work around his AS ... I was really angry and to me, she didn't get how it affected me, the professionals need to understand how it affects both parties, not just one ... The AS unless you're bursting their bubble, do not have a problem, and yet the other partner can be going into anxiety, depression, stressed to the nines, and everybody is saying 'Well I don't know what the problem is, you've got a lovely husband.' Ha.

In Summary

According to Reis et al. (2017) 'perceived understanding is a pervasive, persistent and persuasive force in social life' (p. 15). When people feel understood, it generally benefits the relationship between them; when they feel misunderstood, it generally impairs their relationship (Reis et al., 2017). While NT participants made it clear that they would welcome the opportunity to talk through their difficulties with others, they reported that, ultimately, it proved to be a delicate issue. The lack of understanding, and resulting opinions and conclusions others arrived at, led to mixed reactions, sometimes quite unhelpful. Many NT participants reported that ill-informed people often held them responsible for the relationship's problems. The parental/caretaker role many were required to adopt was found to play some part in maintaining these impressions. The almost exclusive use of instrumental language (that is, factual information used to induce certain actions) that NT participants were mostly required to use, may be misunderstood by others. It was reported that, an appearance of taking care of, or talking to their adult partner/family members with ASC, resembling that of a 'child', was inaccurately regarded by others as condescending behaviour.

Perceptions of mental instability were also frequently reported to develop from incorrect observations of others. Due to unsuccessful attempts at correcting the circular communication debacles, ineffective efforts at making their relationship succeed, and a lack of quantifiable evidence to properly explain their experiences, the majority of NT participants described that family members and other people frequently believed that they were 'crazy'. They described the difficulties and confusion of trying to explain these unspecifiable debacles to others, often gave an appearance of disordered speech and irrational behaviour. A frequent outcome was that, not only did others question their mental health state, but NT participants repeatedly arrived at similar conclusions. Accordingly, symptoms of CP were regularly reported by NT participants and often they abandoned attempts to reach out to others as a result.

The above difficulties developed from the perpetual communication tug-of-war that became the pattern within neurodiverse relationships. At times this communication system cycled in linear ways and at other times in non-linear ways, with neither individual being the victor. The different needs for emotional connectedness, the unsatisfied state of mostly unresolvable differences, the subsequent continuous communication cycles, and the predicament of becoming entangled within the resulting chronic turmoil for people within neurodiverse relationships, when taken together formed multiple difficulties to overcome. Triggered by the communication difficulties, its subsequent prompt dependency cycle, additional cycles and difficulties reaching out to others, three outcomes were identified; the relationship thrives, the relationship survives, or the relationship deteriorates. These outcomes are discussed in the next chapter.

11

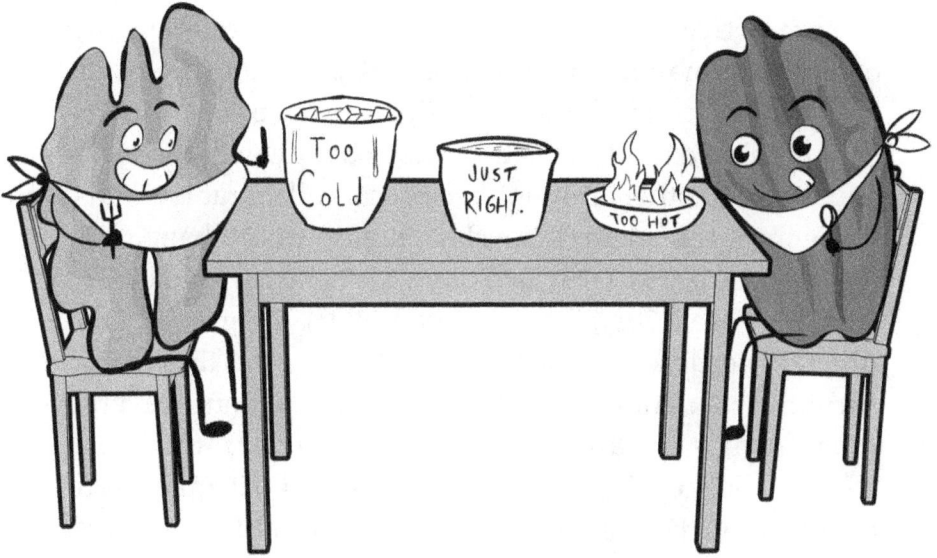

Choices

Have They Gone Nuts?

**'Shared joy is a double joy;
shared sorrow is half a sorrow.'**
Swedish Proverb

Finding the Goldilocks Zone

Interactive behaviour matters greatly to relationship quality (Gottman & Notarius, 2000, 2002). Relationship health is subject to each individual's abilities to adapt and modify their own needs and wants to create a balance with the needs and wants of others through reciprocal collaboration. Thus, while most consider relationships are central to happiness, they are also sources of frustration and challenge (Bodie et al., 2011; Carr et al., 2019; Duck & Wood, 1995). Triggered by the different needs for emotional connectedness and the chronic turmoil from communication difficulties, neurodiverse relationships usually experience more frustrations and more challenges than most. Three potential outcomes were discovered in these studies that arose from identifiable choices.

Some people were thriving. They had found ways to approach their differences in a more positive manner and were prepared to work at ways to resolve their differences. They had come to a decision to do whatever it took to prevail, as best that they could, and make their relationship work. They felt that they were making headway, and although they reported that it was still a work in progress, they were finding their 'just right' in their circumstances. Others were merely surviving. This group felt that the differences were too vast to overcome to a mutually satisfiable manner. While technically still together, they had come to the decision to basically live separate lives. The third group of people had made the decision to give up on their relationship fully. Their relationship was dying or had died. They had found that the problems were insurmountable for them and had decided not to persist any longer.

Choose Thriving

Max (ASC) and Mia (NT) shared how Max had positively responded to the support Mia had provided. He was willing to put into practice the concepts and knowledge he had acquired, rather than remain as mere intellectual understandings. They both shared how these qualities had helped their relationship to grow:

MAX   *I've had a lot of training in terms of how to interact with neurotypicals and a lot of practice so Mia and I are actually a long way down the track ... Mia and I may not be your typical AS-NT relationship ... She's really helped me know what it is to do and so now that I'm actually able to do that, our relationship has improved tremendously.*

MIA   *I'm satisfied in our relationship, particularly in regard to understanding the ways that Max expresses love ... We do share a good connection in that we talk, we spend time together, it's give and take ... I feel a lot of compassion for how difficult life can be for someone with ASD and I have just total respect for Max as a person. He's incredibly humble and open to looking at things in his life that he can do better … It's coming more naturally to him but it's hard … when you have autism … Another thing that makes Max different is his faith … Yeah, I just feel like we do connect during conversations.*

Max also added what it took succeed in a neurodiverse relationship for those with ASC:

It's extra effort … what I've learned and what I know does not come naturally, I have to consciously do it and be aware of my surroundings and people at all times, I just can't do anything automatically.

Similarly, Murray referred to being receptive to talk through miscommunication and putting what he learnt into practice:

We just try and talk about the understanding. Probably the only issues we have is that because I do see things differently, sometimes, we have miscommunication where she thinks the situation means X and I think it means Y and if we don't talk it through then we're not on the same page and there can be issues of confusion. But if we talk, we understand, and I can explain the way I see it and often she will explain to me why that's not the way most people would see it, but at least we're talking through it. Yeah, so over time I've picked up a lot of rules, so particularly when Jane has explained to me 'you shouldn't say this' or 'you should do it that way' or whatever. So, I guess … I've come from being fully clueless to being I now know a lot of them intellectually and therefore I try and practise those, but there are of course still ones I probably don't know so … work in progress.

Choices

The ASC participants who gave accounts of being motivated to learn about, and positively embrace, each other's individual needs, showed that positive outcomes for neurodiverse relationships were possible. When ASC partners/family members were prepared to address their self-protective tendencies and recognise their own lack of communicative ability, they were more inclined to cultivate a positive outlook to their relationship. Rather than escape communication anxieties, or attribute blame to their partner/family members, they were more likely to cope with and work through the demands that communication caused. Phil was trying to find ways to work through all his confusion, unawareness and communicative difficulties to try to make his relationship work:

> We both try to understand the other's feelings, but we don't get it right all the time ... I don't communicate properly with her, no, because I find forming sentences and words very hard ... It used to just make me freeze ... because everything was happening too fast ... I am slowly learning to be a bit better at that and not freeze and just say 'Woo, I need time to think, I need time to catch up.' I have learned how to do that.

Mark, as well, by recognising his position, was trying to work through the communication problems with Kay rather than escape or blame:

> Our relationship? On the whole I think it's a very, very close, loving relationship. It's probably the closest relationship that I have ever had in my life, but there are elements of occasions where things do go sort of off the rails a bit, due to my lack of social skills, my lack of reading emotions, and not being

able to empathise very well at all. So, there are things that I do that drive her out of her tree.

Daniel showed a willingness to learn about his autism, and learn from his partner:

Cathy is good at establishing relationships and works hard at it. We have discovered autism together. She is sympathetic, but her theory of mind doesn't quite grasp the autistic model … We work hard at being good to each other … What I know of kindness I have learned from Cathy.

Similarly, Terry revealed that an awareness of the diagnosis and a willingness to learn from his partner had helped him:

Well, the expectation that I've grown to understand is that I need to actually consciously spend more time with Kim and to further develop my communication skills … I know Kim is so different to me in communication skills, but luckily, she's quite strong and quite often reminds me that … my communication skills [need] improving … I think I'm doing a lot better than I used to, and being aware of the various conditions that I have, Asperger's diagnosis from about six or seven years ago.

Barry commended his wife's ability to turn away his anger:

I might say silly things … more irrational maybe. Hope doesn't ever say anything irrational by the way; she doesn't reflect back; she just seems to absorb it like a stealth plane. It doesn't bounce the radar back, ha, ha … and in a way I suppose, like I say, 'A quiet word turns away anger', so it does work.

Choices

Richard recognised that working together and finding the positives was the way forward:

> *Realising something's not there ... and trying to fix it. We're trying to work in the right direction. We don't want to sort of end up in separation ... There's a lot of good things ... Yes, we've had disagreements, and yes, we realise the relationship should be better, but as I say, talking to you, that's what we're trying to get some things down to help make it work.*

Malcolm's comment sums up the ASC-NT communicative dilemma:

> *Grace says it's the hardest and the most rewarding relationship that she has ever had. Like, to have an Aspie, the experiences that we have, and the qualities are very worthwhile, and yet, it is frustration beyond frustration.*

Mary decided a family meeting was the way to improve understanding:

> *And we had a family meeting over this actually because I needed for everyone to understand. And this was after the Asperger's diagnosis because we were trying to help limit the amount of distress in communication ... [be]cause I'm quite literal.*

Like ASC participants, many NT participants shared that recognition and acceptance of the diagnosis from both sides made a significant difference to their relationship. Sophie stated this was the case for her:

> *He recently had his aha moment last year in realising he has Asperger's Syndrome. I am incredibly expressive with my*

emotions, and he is able to express himself well too … The key to making this work between us is clear communication and honesty from both sides. That also means being honest about emotional states and communicating them to each other. This goes for negative emotions as well as positive. We have to be able to tell each other we do not like an action, just as much as if we liked another.

Likewise, Winnie described how awareness of the diagnosis can be transforming:

Well, I think from what the women that I have read about, the women that I have met in the group, I am just amazed by (a) their resilience and (b) persistence too, and the hard work they put into learn[ing] and the efforts to make the relationship work and to teach themselves about the condition rather than just walk away.

Ruth described how their relationship had improved:

We have made progress … Now, he seems to realise that what I say IS valid or important, more often than he used to. I feel like I'm starting to matter more, which is a step in the right direction.

Even while appreciating her partner's limitations, Laura shared how cherishing each other, can make a big difference:

He once or twice has indicated that I, and the home I have created for him, has saved him from despair, but he avoids emotional discussions.

An anonymous comment from an NT survey respondent revealed that understanding is key to findings solutions:

I study Psychology and Criminology, so I do have an understanding of their inability to show empathy and problem-solve and negotiate. I will just accept that they will not apologise and move on, but it does not take away the hurt that I felt from being treated that way. I am fortunate that I can understand them, though, as it helps me deal with it better. I do miss the deep and meaningful conversations, but again understand the difficulties. My husband and I have been to some counselling over the years, and he does try hard. We have recently been using the John Gottman program on using empathy, and he has been achieving some great results learning how to empathise. When something happens, he has to try and recognise the emotion in that person and then say, 'I think you're feeling ... '. It also helps the kids try and express their feelings as well. We have a son on the spectrum and our daughter has features.

Choose Surviving

Many participants felt that the differences were insurmountable for them, so they had found ways to live separate lives, while still together. Several participants reported that they had become more like housemates behind closed doors while acting and looking like a 'normal relationship' in public. A few participants reported that they had become resigned to their current situation and were trying to make their relationship tolerable as best they could, while others had completely disconnected. Not many ASC participants discussed these aspects, however, a few identified some of the decisions they had made to survive living the differences alone together:

SAMUEL   *We are simply companions ... We do pretty much our own thing apart from the odd thing together. We travel together ... but affection is really just making each other a cup of tea and coffee and sitting and chatting together, that's about it really.*

DANIEL   *We've had 20 years of practice at getting along. There is something in my tone or look occasionally that triggers fight or flight in Cathy. I've never managed to pin it down.*

EDITH   *First of all they've got to recognise that you actually do have some difficulties that are hardwired not soft wired and that you also have to have the opportunity to work through things in different ways which means that they have to be more flexible and perhaps less judgemental.*

In contrast, NT participants had much to say about surviving a relationship that was not as they imagined. Many described that after considerable effort, the strain of trying to make their expectations materialise caused many to emotionally withdraw from the relationship:

WANDA   *I've kind of given up ... I think I've kind of worn myself out. I'm a bit blasé I'm sorry, you can add that to the data, I guess ... Yeah, I've sort of reached that point of not being hurt anymore and trying not to expect anything and I don't have the answers.*

MAGGIE *I won't put myself forward anymore and share as much as I would like to share with him because of his reaction and his unknowing of how to deal with it on an emotional level ... people say, 'Oh look, you've just got to get all your needs met somewhere else with your friends' ... and I thought to myself 'but that's not a marriage'.*

DIANNE *Our relationship is very much, I think two people boarding in the same house ... My two boys were married ... since they left home ... the relationship became more strained. Because you expect then, that when you are on your own, you will have more time for one another. And I guess that realisation and the expectation from me and the fact that there wasn't really a sharing relationship it was more of ... I feel like his carer these days rather than his partner.*

FIONA *There is no affection. There is no feeling of belonging. After the initial phase of courtship, right that's done, put that away, on with the next part of life, which doesn't involve any affection, or feeling part of a relationship ... just sort of two people: cohabiting.*

TRACY *I don't feel like expressing warmth or affection anymore because there is no more affection*

> *… I don't think he notices. Of course, I have given up now. I just try and get on with my life and look after my children. I have also made friendships a priority, seeking emotional closeness with people of the same sex, good friends. I miss the closeness with a husband because it has a physical side to it, but I have a lot of single friends who are not sexually active either, so I know it's possible. It's just a lot more painful when you are married.*

An anonymous comment from an NT survey respondent gave a powerful rendition of some of the difficulties of scarcely surviving in this way:

> *We have experienced huge difficulties over our marriage. I thought I was the problem so have striven endlessly to improve things. I'm a counsellor by training. Now since the diagnosis I find it easier, as I have an explanation, however I hate the way it is me who polices, emotional gate keeps and mothers the relationship. My only MO now, is to have a largely separate existence where I am nurtured by others, and I do not look to him for any emotional support. We are now just flatmates instead of lovers. Part of this was bought on by his infidelities (one of 15 years duration) resulting in a separation of 15 months. He is emotionally naive and seemingly unaware of his contribution to the problem. One large change, however is, he has learned to say 'Sorry' and that has helped me adjust. It has been very, very hard work. I have to work at developing a life that is separate to his, in order to stay sane. It is so sad to have to acknowledge 'He is a blind man in a sighted*

world, and he has kicked his guide dog in the teeth.' I'm staying, because financially I would be much worse off if separated, however, accepting that this is all there is, is tough. The rest of our friends cannot see the problem, as he is very skilled at morphing into whatever is required; I describe him as an 'amoeba'. Get him alone and try to solve an issue and then you realise how convoluted his thinking is. He is gentle and described as a lovely man – yes, until you get to know him! He is skilled at reflecting whatever is going on around him, but has no ideas or opinions of his own, merely deflecting what others say, by being agreeable. What I call 'a hollow man'. Keep up the good work; this is a maddening issue.

Similar comments from NT survey respondents illustrates similar feelings; the difficulties of merely surviving, the relief felt when finally having an answer, and the despair felt when unable to find ways to rectify or improve the situation:

After years of frustration a therapist finally diagnosed my spouse with Asperger's and that has made a very big difference in what I expect in our relationship. The anxiety level has decreased for both of us. I have stopped expecting a NT relationship and look for the good qualities that are in our relationship.

My husband has Asperger's ... It's only those that have experienced what I'm going through, that will understand. There's always going to be that longing for what will never be ... that longing for a life that only exists in fairy tales. What must it be like? To have a relationship with someone who 'gets you', to 'connect'. I can only imagine. But I mustn't waste time wistfully wishing for something, as I know it's beyond him to 'get' me. I have an enviable life. He definitely loves me, about that I have no doubt, and he is so devoted, it's just something ... that's difficult to explain unless you've been there or are there.

Choose Dying

Many participants lamented the demise of the relationship that they had hoped for but had to come to the realisation that it was not an option for them. As a result, some decided to solve the problem by remaining in the same house, but live separate lives, others lived in separate houses and continued to see each other, while a few decided that divorce was the only option. Although, a few participants in the study had decided to completely leave their relationship, anecdotal evidence suggests that it is a rare occurrence for those within neurodiverse relationships to divorce. The main reason appears to be that, when awareness of the condition occurs, and understanding grows, accommodation of the condition follows. Sometimes, however, understanding occurs too late to save the relationship. Sharon (ASC), disclosed that her need for solitude ended her marriage:

He understood that I needed some level of solitude, but that took a toll in the marriage eventually.

She went on to give her thoughts on how to save neurodiverse relationships:

For any relationship to stay strong and go far, they must be allowed to be themselves – AS or NT – and still enjoy the relationship.

Choices

Many NT participants reported that they attempted to find unconventional solutions if conventional ones were not an option for them. Tracy had found that a solution for her was to use an empty room in her house:

I just stop talking and leave. I need to protect myself. We now have an empty room in the house, and I can withdraw there.

Ronda shared that, while they now lived in separate houses and in different areas of the country, she was prepared to be her ex-husband's caretaker for life:

I have completely abandoned any hope of ever having an intimate partner, an intimate companion with whom I would have an emotional connection ... The divorce and the annulment came basically to ratify an already existing situation forever ... I have accepted freely willingly and 100% without any reserve to be his caretaker for life, for the rest of his life, if necessary, if he doesn't go on to remarry ... Practically every day, we're very happy to see each other on Skype. We share our news, what's going on in our lives ... because I find that it's important to just continue to be present because I just recently moved, three weeks ago, to a different state.

However, Haley reported that her marriage had ended a few weeks prior to the interview:

I really hope you do get some answers out of it ... how to actually deal with it ... [be]cause, I've ended up, I've left. We've been gone now for about five weeks... I just said, 'Look I'm not happy, I look at you and I think you're not happy as well.' ... Like in the end we just stopped talking.

Have They Gone Nuts?

An anonymous comment from NT survey respondent described how their relationship had deteriorated over time:

Our relationship would improve if my partner were capable of seeing beyond his own experience and point of view. Our relationship would improve if my partner knew how to validate my experiences and values. Our relationship would improve if my partner knew how to respond to my needs instead of setting the pace of the relationship by his own standards of needs and satisfaction. Our relationship would improve if my partner would respect my communicational, emotional and empathetic abilities and trust that I can see many things he cannot. Our relationship would improve if my partner took seriously the impact his Asperger's has on our life, our relationship, our intimacy, and my life as a practically married-but-single-parent. Our relationship would improve if my partner learned how to give meaningful verbal praise and recognition on a regular basis. Our relationship would improve if my partner trusted my opinions and experiences as a parent.

In Summary

Contrasts are a part of life and, while most consider relationships as central to happiness, relationships are also sources of frustration and challenge (Carr et al., 2019). The three potential outcomes observed for neurodiverse relationships, triggered by the different needs for emotional connectedness, the unsatisfied state of the relentless differences, and the subsequent continuous communication cycles, while mainly discouraging, also indicated some encouraging results.

Thriving
Although limited, outcomes for these relationships can be positive. When able to access appropriate support, that is, support from people knowledgeable in the area of ASC, together with an acceptance of the diagnosis from both parties, the likelihood of a positive outcome can be improved (Attwood, 2015; Moreno et al., 2012). Additional aspects that can improve the prospect of a positive outcome were in the areas of knowledge, awareness and learning. Important aspects that were observed to encourage promising results were: gaining neurodiversity knowledge and understanding; the ability to apply a constructive mindset; and the motivation for both parties to learn about the needs of each and apply the information gained.

Surviving
The majority of ASC and NT participants felt that the differences, found within neurodiverse relationships, were often insurmountable. When matters become unmanageable, the inability of each person within the relationship to regard themselves as part of a collective unit, and instead, live parallel disconnected lives (Bentley, 2007), became an inescapable pattern. A developing lack of interest in each other, a perpetual unresponsiveness toward each other, and a progression of indifference and emotional withdrawal from each other, appeared to be the main results from living within the limitations of this pattern. Exhibiting a non-authentic life that looked standard on the outside, but non-standard on the inside, seemed to become the custom for this

group of participants, with many reporting that they were living more like disconnected housemates than partners or close family members.

Deteriorating

Sometimes destructive results occur and outcomes can, therefore, be undesirable. Surprisingly, this outcome was not a frequent finding. Awareness of the autism spectrum can buffer some of the negative effects of resultant difficulties. Sometimes, however, awareness occurs too late to save the relationship. Participants who were in this group expressed anguish and grief over the demise of the relationship that they had hoped for but realised was not an option for them. As a result, some decided to solve the problem by remaining in the same house while living completely separate lives. Others lived in separate houses and continued seeing each other from time to time, whereas a few decided that divorce and/or complete separation was the only option.

In the final chapter, the key messages of the book are revealed, along with identifiable solutions and a model that illustrates the dynamic communication interplay between people in neurodiverse relationships.

12

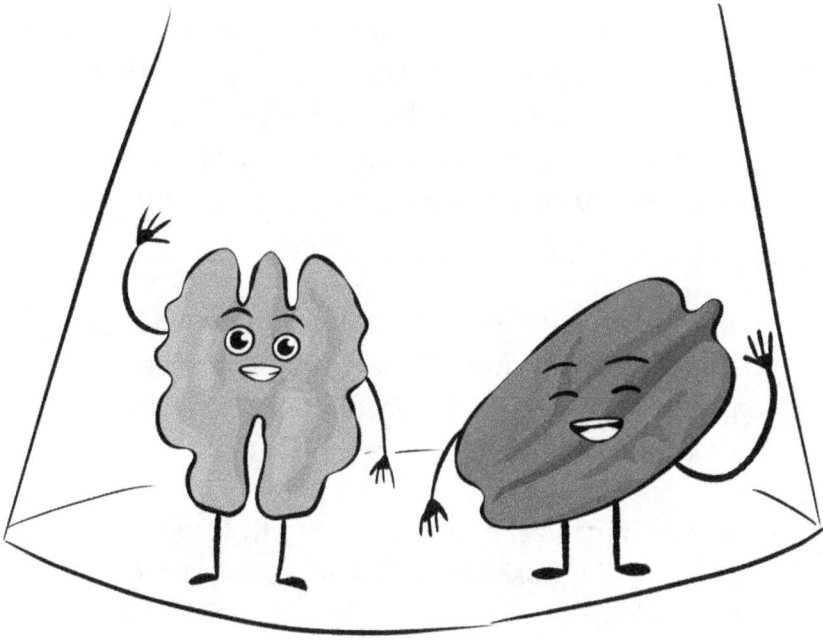

Nuts and Bolts

Have They Gone Nuts?

'A dialogue is not made up of two monologues.'
Howard E. Short,
United Church Herald, Vol. 10, 1967

The Key Message

Derived from my years of study and presented through the voices of people in neurodiverse relationships, the key message of this book is that, although there are many difficulties to overcome, there are identifiable actions that people can take to ensure a more positive outcome.

To encourage a potential to thrive in a neurodiverse relationship and reduce the negative influences of the complex system of circular conversations found in these studies it is essential to:

- Be willing to accept and willing to learn about an ASC diagnosis, even if self-diagnosed. (That means both of you: the person with ASC and the NT person). Read everything. Learn everything. Become your own guru.

- Be willing to gain neurodiversity knowledge and learn about each other's differences. (i.e. what it means to be neurotypical if you are autistic, and what it means to be autistic if you are neurotypical).

- Tackle the relationship with a constructive mindset. Continually look for ways to improve things from your position. Don't wait for the other. Make it a priority.

- Understand that typical counselling will never suffice. Support given from a lack of appropriate knowledge is not support. It does more harm than good. If you find that you need help, locate appropriate support (i.e. support from people knowledgeable in neurodiverse relationships). There are also many great resources that can be found on the internet.

- Most importantly, be motivated to learn about, nurture and support each individual's needs. Your spouse and your family are the most important people in the world. Your words and your behaviour need to reflect that fact.

Illuminating the Message

The model (see Appendix 1), developed in these studies, while showing many negative outcomes, also shows the potential for positive outcomes that are useful for consideration for people in neurodiverse relationships, for people who develop and deliver counselling programs, and for researchers in this area of study. Commencing with the need NT individuals have of healthy reciprocal relationships by means of deep conversation, companionship and intimacy, the model illustrates that this need was often thwarted by the social interaction difficulties experienced with their

ASC partners/family members. Alternatively, attributable to these difficulties, adults with ASC often need to socially disengage and find a place of solitude and refuge in non-social activities to achieve respite from their interaction challenges. The model reveals that two trajectories follow. The social interaction difficulties experienced by autistic adults trigger NT adults to prompt to improve interaction, encourage involvement and meet their need for a healthy reciprocal relationship. Sometimes, the actions prompted are accomplished. Frequently, however, partners/family members with ASC remain unresponsive and/or avoid the prompts. This avoidance regularly causes an increase in prompting. Intermittent schedules of reinforcement are very resistant to extinction. Therefore, the partial effectiveness of the prompts set in motion a process of oscillation between the prompting behaviour of NT adults and the avoidance, and/or response behaviours of ASC adults which, in turn, intensified the prompting behaviour of NT adults. The model illustrates how this oscillation activated the formation of an intertwined cycle of prompting with prompt dependency and/or self-protectiveness.

The second pathway arises from the need that those with ASC had of social disengagement. This path converges with and influences, both these cycles. Effects such as, a lack of asking questions, misinterpreting actions and inaccurate assumptions furthers a lack of engagement with conversations, which similarly, furthers the oscillation between prompting and self-protective behaviour and/or dependency on prompts. The intensification of these intertwined behaviours shapes the development of a parental/caretaker role for NT adults with neither group of people succeeding in attainment of their needs.

The model illustrates that added interaction cycles result from the power struggle of unresolved needs attainment. These cycles, the imitating normalcy cycle, the stonewalling cycle, the seeking help cycle and the loss of sense of self cycle, all cycled in the background and alongside the intertwined prompt dependency cycle and self-protective cycle, while also converging with and influencing both cycles. The three possible outcomes of these interaction cycles are also illustrated.

Appendix 1: Prompt Dependency Cycle with Interwoven Additional Cycles and Potential Outcomes (over page)

Have They Gone Nuts?

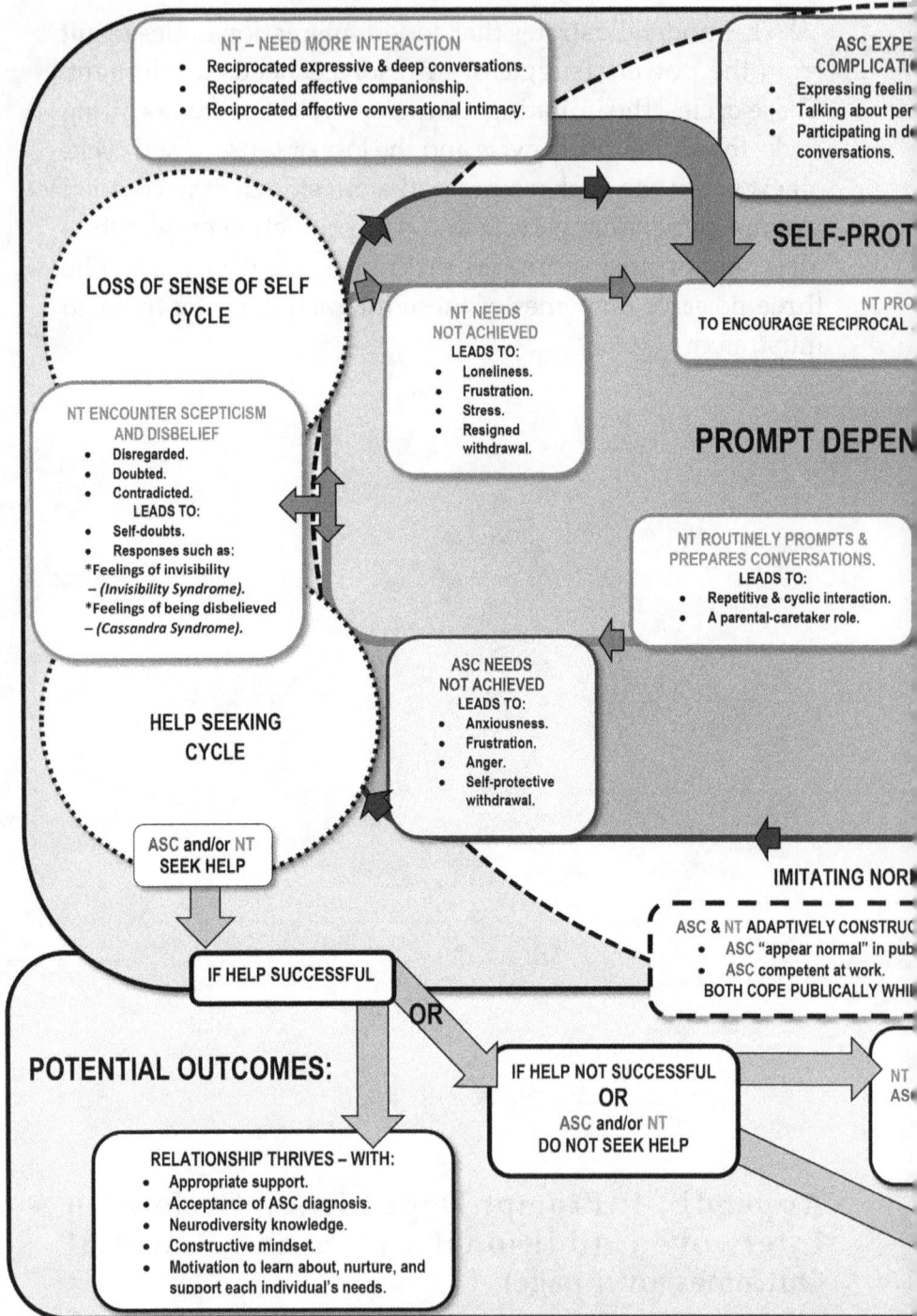

NT – NEED MORE INTERACTION
- Reciprocated expressive & deep conversations.
- Reciprocated affective companionship.
- Reciprocated affective conversational intimacy.

**ASC EXPE
COMPLICATI**
- Expressing feelin
- Talking about per
- Participating in de
conversations.

SELF-PROT

**LOSS OF SENSE OF SELF
CYCLE**

**NT NEEDS
NOT ACHIEVED
LEADS TO:**
- Loneliness.
- Frustration.
- Stress.
- Resigned withdrawal.

NT PRO
TO ENCOURAGE RECIPROCAL

PROMPT DEPEN

**NT ENCOUNTER SCEPTICISM
AND DISBELIEF**
- Disregarded.
- Doubted.
- Contradicted.
LEADS TO:
- Self-doubts.
- Responses such as:
*Feelings of invisibility
– *(Invisibility Syndrome).*
*Feelings of being disbelieved
– *(Cassandra Syndrome).*

**NT ROUTINELY PROMPTS &
PREPARES CONVERSATIONS.
LEADS TO:**
- Repetitive & cyclic interaction.
- A parental-caretaker role.

**ASC NEEDS
NOT ACHIEVED
LEADS TO:**
- Anxiousness.
- Frustration.
- Anger.
- Self-protective withdrawal.

**HELP SEEKING
CYCLE**

**ASC and/or NT
SEEK HELP**

IMITATING NOR

ASC & NT ADAPTIVELY CONSTRUC
- ASC "appear normal" in pub
- ASC competent at work.
BOTH COPE PUBLICALLY WHI

IF HELP SUCCESSFUL

OR

**IF HELP NOT SUCCESSFUL
OR
ASC and/or NT
DO NOT SEEK HELP**

NT
AS

POTENTIAL OUTCOMES:

RELATIONSHIP THRIVES – WITH:
- Appropriate support.
- Acceptance of ASC diagnosis.
- Neurodiversity knowledge.
- Constructive mindset.
- Motivation to learn about, nurture, and support each individual's needs.

**XPERIENCE
ATIONS WITH:**
- elings and emotions.
- personal matters.
- in deep and meaningful
- s.

LEADS TO:

ASC – NEED LESS INTERACTION
- Company without expressive & deep conversations.
- Solitude to relieve tensions.
- Refuge in special interests.

OTECTIVE CYCLE

ASC RESPONDS TO NT PROMPTS.

OR

ASC AVOIDS NT PROMPTS.
Using stonewalling behaviours:
- Defensiveness.
- Shutting down.
- Verbal aggression.

PROMPT
AL AFFECTION & CONNECTION.

ENDENCY CYCLE

**NT INTENSIFY PROMPTS
DUE TO SUCCESS OR TO SOLVE ASC AVOIDANCE.**

**NT RESPONSE
DUE TO INTERMITTENT SUCCESS**
- Repeatedly prompt.

ASC RESPONSE
- Interaction anxiety
- Unresponsiveness
- Lack of asking questions.
- Misinterpreting actions.
- Inaccurate assumptions.

INFORMING:
- Expectations.
- Decisions.
- Conclusions.
- The formation of rules.
- Level of cooperation.
- Lack of self-initiation.
- Lack of insight.
- Lack of motivation.

ASC INTERPRETATIONS AND REACTIONS
LEADS TO:
- Prompt dependency AND/OR Prompt avoidance.
- Unresponsiveness.
- Stonewalling behaviour.
- Inflexible behaviour.

STONEWALLING CYCLE

ORMALCY CYCLE

RUCT NORMALCY IN PUBLIC SINCE
public.

VHILE LIVING PARALLEL LIVES.

RELATIONSHIP SURVIVES – ALTHOUGH:
NT – Unreciprocated affection triggers a loss of interest for affection.
ASC – Increased detachment.
- Both withdraw from the relationship.
- A hidden reality.
- Living alone together.

RELATIONSHIP DETERIORATES – LEADING TO:
- Relationship breaks down.
- Separation.
- Divorce.

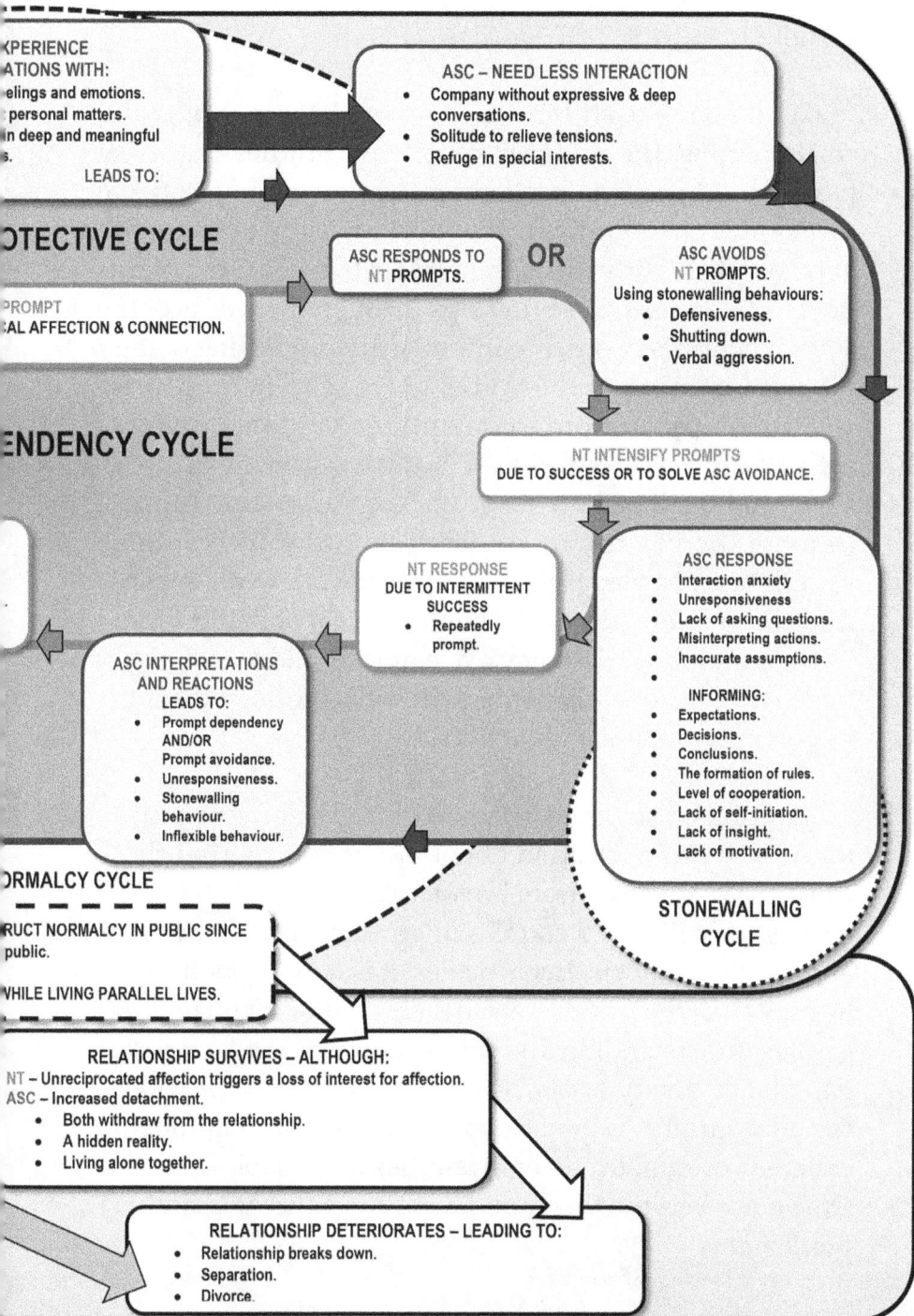

For colour version: https://bronwilson.com/model/

Final Thoughts

While there is still much to learn about neurodiverse relationships, the findings of the two studies highlight participants' perspectives concerning the communicational difficulties that adults in these relationships experience and how these difficulties shape their lives. The aim of this book is to present these findings through the words of the 400 participants in order to improve understanding of their reality. Listening to the voices of those in neurodiverse relationships, not only contributes valuable insights into their lived experience but also gives others an understanding of how to provide comfort and support to them. By improving understanding of their unique experiences, opportunities are provided to work towards finding solutions to overcome the effects of being caught in the prompt dependency cycle and its additional cycles from within the relationship, while also giving others the opportunity to assist from outside.

Findings also stress the need for greater community awareness and education about issues confronting those in neurodiverse relationships to reduce the distress felt by these families and couples in general, and NT partners and family members, in particular. It is hoped that through hearing from the participants in these studies, it will promote greater understanding and aid in bridging the knowledge gap that currently exists between many service providers, the community in general, and the unique relationship experiences of neurodiverse families and couples. Sabrina (NT) conveyed the viewpoint of most of the ASC and NT participants:

Nuts and Bolts

*Since so many of these relationship issues naturally end up
in marriage counselling ... there needs to be a better job done
in the education of psychologists, social workers ... so that
they don't inflict the traditional counselling on [them] ...
It's never going to work, and it's just going to cause more
harm than good.*

The next book in the *Have They Gone Nuts?* series addresses Sabrina's concerns. Through the participants' narratives, we discover what takes place when they reach out to others to access support and/or services. Since many clinicians and counsellors went through their education at a time when the autism spectrum was relatively unknown, the participants share how a lack of professional and community knowledge impacts on their abilities to access appropriate professional help. They also share what it is like coming to terms with a realisation of autism in later life and what they want their family and friends to know. Alongside this we hear their thoughts and ideas on ways to advance their needs, increase professional and community understanding and build more positive perspectives of neurodiverse relationships, both from the the inside and the outside of these unique relationships. They also reveal various constructive ways forward that they have uncovered for themselves.

In the third book of the series, the participants convey a strong message of hope for future directions and discuss what they would like researchers, academics, healthcare providers and policy makers to know. Look out for the next two books in this series to further enhance your understanding of the neurodiverse experience from the inside.

About the Author

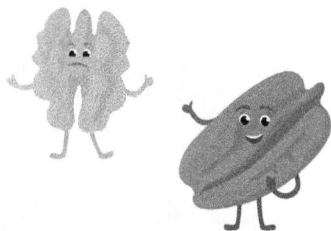

Bronwyn Wilson lives in a small beachside town in Western Australia, after moving from Queensland for her husband's work. Following a career in teaching she embarked on research, completing a PhD thesis at Edith Cowan University, Perth, Western Australia, researching the communication difficulties that can occur within the close relationships of adults with ASD Level 1 (Asperger's Syndrome). Bronwyn also holds a Master of Special Education, obtained from Griffith University, Brisbane, and a Bachelor of Education, obtained from James Cook University, Townsville.

She has published peer-reviewed papers and presented at the 5th Asia Pacific Autism Conference in 2017 held at the International Convention Centre in Sydney, and at the 5th World Autism Conference, Houston, Texas, USA in 2018. Today, Bronwyn works as an online sessional tutor at Edith Cowan University while also authoring books and journal articles. She enjoys swimming most days, sewing

Have They Gone Nuts?

and decorating her home, along with watching the boats go past, listening to the waves and enjoying the ocean views from her verandah.

References

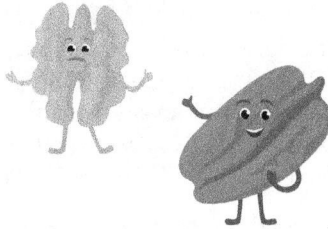

Akshoomoff, N., Pierce, K., & Courchesne, E. (2002). The neurobiological basis of autism from a developmental perspective. *Development and Psychopathology, 14*, 613–634. https://doi.org/10.1017.S0954579402003115

Arad, P., Shechtman, Z., & Attwood, T. (2022). Physical and mental wellbeing of women in neurodiverse relationships: A comparative study. *Journal of Psychology & Psychotherapy, 12*(1), 1-9.

Arioli, M., Crespi, C., & Canessa, N. (2018). Social cognition through the lens of cognitive and clinical neuroscience. *BioMed Research International*, 4283427. https://doi.org/10.1155/2018/4283427

Aston, M. (2001). *The other half of Asperger Syndrome: A guide to living in a relationship with a partner who has Asperger Syndrome*. The National Autistic Society.

Aston, M. (2003). *Aspergers in love. Couple relationships and family affairs*. Jessica Kingsley Publishers.

Attwood, T. (2015). *The complete guide to Asperger's Syndrome* (Revised ed.). Jessica Kingsley Publishers.

Baez, S., & Ibanez, A. (2014). The effects of context processing on social cognition impairments in adults with Asperger's syndrome. *Frontiers in Neuroscience*, n/a. https://doi.org/10.3389/fnins.2014.00270

Baron-Cohen, S. (1997). *Mindblindness. An essay on autism and theory of mind*. The MIT Press.

Baron-Cohen, S. (2008). Theories of the autistic mind. *Psychologist, 21*(2), 112–116.

Baumeister, R. F., & Leary, M. R. (1995). The need to belong: Desire for interpersonal attachments as a fundamental human motivation. *Psychological Bulletin, 117*(3), 497–529. https://doi.org/10.1037/0033-2909.117.3.497

Benning, S. D., Kovac, M., Campbell, A., Miller, S., Hanna, E. K., Damiano, C. R., Sabatino-DiCriscio, A., Turner-Brown, L., Sasson, N. J., Aaron, R. V., Kinard, J., & Dichter, G. S. (2016). Late positive potential ERP responses to social and nonsocial stimuli in youth with autism spectrum disorder. *Journal of Autism and Developmental Disorders, 46*(9), 3068–3077. https://doi.org/10.1007/s10803-016-2845-y

Bentley, K. (2007). *Alone together: Making an Asperger marriage work.* Jessica Kingsley Publishers.

Bodie, G. D., Burleson, B. R., Holmstrom, A. J., McCullough, J. D., Rack, J. J., Hanasono, L. K., & Rosier, J. G. (2011). Effects of cognitive complexity and emotional upset on processing supportive messages: Two tests of a dual-process theory of supportive communication outcomes. *Human Communication Research, 37*(3), 350–376. https://doi.org/10.1111/j.1468-2958.2011.01405.x

Bostock-Ling, J. S. (2017). *Life satisfaction of neurotypical women in intimate relationship with a partner who has Asperger's Syndrome: An exploratory study.* University of Sydney.

Bottini, S. (2018). Social reward processing in individuals with autism spectrum disorder: A systematic review of the social motivation hypothesis. *Research in Autism Spectrum Disorders, 45*(29), 9–26.

Brown, L. H., Silvia, P. J., Myin-Germeys, I., & Kwapil, T. R. (2007). When the need to belong goes wrong: The expression of social anhedonia and social anxiety in daily life. *Psychological Science, 18*(9), 778–782.

Bryan, L. C., & Gast, D. L. (2000). Teaching on-task and on-schedule behaviours to high-functioning children with autism via picture activity schedules. *Journal of Autism and Developmental Disorders, 30*(6), 553–567. https://doi.org/10.1023/a:1005687310346

Burleson, B. R. (2003). The experience and effects of emotional support: What the study of cultural and gender differences can tell us about close relationships, emotion, and interpersonal communication. *Personal Relationships, 10*(1), 1–23. https://doi.org/10.1111/1475-6811.00033

References

Burleson, B. R. (2009). Understanding the outcomes of supportive communication: A dual-process approach. *Journal of Social and Personal Relationships, 26*(1), 21–38. http://spr.sagepub.com.ezproxy.ecu.edu.au/content/26/1/21

Butler, E. A., & Randall, A. K. (2013). Emotional coregulation in close relationships. *Emotion Review, 5*(2), 202–210. https://doi.org/10.1177/1754073912451630

Carr, D., Cornman, J. C., & Freedman, V. A. (2019). Do family relationships buffer the impact of disability on older adults' daily mood? An exploration of gender and marital status differences. *Journal of Marriage and Family, 81*(3), 729–746. https://doi.org/10.1111/jomf.12557

Caruana, N., McArthur, G., Woolgar, A., & Brock, J. (2017). Simulating social interactions for the experimental investigation of joint attention. *Neuroscience & Biobehavioral Reviews, 74*(Part A), 115–125. https://doi.org/https://doi.org/10.1016/j.neubiorev.2016.12.022

Casanova, E. L., & Casanova, M. F. (2019). *Defining autism: A guide to brain, biology, and behavior.* Jessica Kingsley Publishers. https://search.ebscohost.com/login.aspx?direct=true&scope=site&db=nlebk&db=nlabk&AN=1927427

Craig, J., & Baron-Cohen, S. (1999). Creativity and Imagination in Autism and Asperger Syndrome. *Journal of Autism and Developmental Disorders, 29*(4), 319–326. https://doi.org/10.1023/A:1022163403479

Deisinger, J. A. (2011). History of autism spectrum disorders. In A. Rotatori (Ed.), *History of Special Education* (Vol. 21, pp. 237–267). Emerald Group Publishing Limited.

Derlega, V. J. (2013). *Communication, intimacy, and close relationships.* Elsevier.

Domire, S. C., & Wolfe, P. (2014). Effects of video prompting techniques on teaching daily living skills to children with Autism Spectrum Disorders: A review. *Research & Practice for Persons with Severe Disabilities, 39*(3), 211–226. https://doi.org/10.1177/1540796914555578

Dubin, N. (2009). *Asperger Syndrome and anxiety.* Jessica Kingsley Publishers.

Duck, S., & Wood, J. T. (1995). For better, for worse, for richer, for poorer: The rough and the smooth of relationships. In *Confronting relationship challenges.* SAGE Publications, Inc. https://doi.org/10.4135/9781483327181

Egan, V., & Linenberg, O. (2019). The measurement of adult pathological demand avoidance traits. *Journal of Autism and Developmental Disorders, 49*(2), 481–494. https://doi.org/10.1007/s10803-018-3722-7

Eid, P., & Boucher, S. (2012). Alexithymia and dyadic adjustment in intimate relationships: Analyses using the actor partner interdependence model. *Journal of Social and Clinical Psychology, 31*(10), 1095–1111. https://doi.org/http://dx.doi.org/101521jscp201231101095

Garris, B. R., & Weber, A. J. (2018). Relationships influence health: Family theory in health-care research. *Journal of Family Theory & Review, 10*(4), 712–734. https://doi.org/10.1111/jftr.12294

Gillberg, C., Gillberg, I. C., Thompson, L., Biskupsto, R., & Billstedt, E. (2015). Extreme ("pathological") demand avoidance in autism: a general population study in the Faroe Islands. *European Child & Adolescent Psychiatry, 24*(8), 979–984. https://doi.org/10.1007/s00787-014-0647-3

Gillespie-Smith, K., Ballantyne, C., Branigan, H. P., Turk, D. J., & Cunningham, S. J. (2018). The I in autism: Severity and social functioning in autism are related to self-processing. *British Journal of Developmental Psychology, 36*(1), 127–141. https://doi.org/10.1111/bjdp.12219

Gottman, J. (1993). The roles of conflict engagement, escalation, and avoidance in marital interaction: a longitudinal view of five types of couples. *Journal of Consulting and Clinical Psychology, 61*(1), 6.

Gottman, J., & Gottman, J. (2017). The natural principles of love. *Journal of Family Theory & Review, 9*(1), 7–26. https://doi.org/10.1111/jftr.12182

Gottman, J., & Notarius, C. I. (2000). Decade review: Observing marital interaction. *Journal of Marriage and the Family, 62*(4), 927–947.

Gottman, J., & Notarius, C. I. (2002). Marital research in the 20th century and a research agenda for the 21st century. *Family Process, 41*(2), 159–197. https://doi.org/10.1111/j.1545-5300.2002.41203.x

Griffin, C., Lombardo, M. V., & Auyeung, B. (2016). Alexithymia in children with and without autism spectrum disorders. *Autism Research, 9*(7), 773–780.

Grigg, C. (2012). *ASPIA's handbook for partner support: A collection of ASPIA's best information for the support of partners of adults with Asperger's Syndrome.* Carol Grigg. www.aspia.org.au

Han, G. T., Tomarken, A. J., & Gotham, K. O. (2019). Social and nonsocial reward moderate the relation between autism symptoms and loneliness

References

in adults with ASD, depression, and controls. *Autism Research, 12*(6), 884–896. https://doi.org/10.1002/aur.2088

Harris, J. (2018). Leo Kanner and autism: a 75-year perspective. *International Review of Psychiatry, 30*(1), 3–17. https://doi.org/10.1080/09540261.2018.1455646

Heller, J. (1961). *Catch-22.* Jonathon Cape.

Hesse, C. (2020). Affection deprivation in marital relationships: An actor-partner interdependence mediation analysis. *Journal of Social and Personal Relationships, 37*(3), 965–985. https://doi.org/10.1177/0265407519883697

Hickey, A., Crabtree, J., & Stott, J. (2017). 'Suddenly the first fifty years of my life made sense': Experiences of older people with autism. *Autism, 0*(0), 1362361316680914. https://doi.org/doi:10.1177/1362361316680914

Hull, L., Petrides, K. V., Allison, C., Smith, P., Baron-Cohen, S., Lai, M.-C., & Mandy, W. (2017). "Putting on my best normal": Social camouflaging in adults with autism spectrum conditions. *Journal of Autism and Developmental Disorders, 47*(8), 2519–2534.

Jacobs, B. (2006). *Loving Mr Spock. Undertsanding an aloof lover. Could it be Asperger's Syndrome?.* Jessica Kingsley Publishers.

Jennings, S. (2005). Autism in children and parents: unique considerations for family court professionals. *Family Court Review, 43*(4), 582–595.

Lai, M.-C., & Baron-Cohen, S. (2015). Identifying the lost generation of adults with autism spectrum conditions. *The Lancet Psychiatry, 2*(11), 1013–1027.

Lasser, J., & Corley, K. (2008). Constructing normalcy: a qualitative study of parenting children with Asperger's Disorder. *Educational Psychology in Practice, 24*(4), 335–346. https://doi.org/10.1080/02667360802488773

Laurenceau, J.-P., Pietromonaco, P. R., & Barrett, L. F. (1998). Intimacy as an interpersonal process: the importance of self-disclosure, partner disclosure, and perceived partner responsiveness in interpersonal exchanges. *Journal of Personality and Social Psychology, 74*(5), 1238–1251.

Lehnhardt, F.-G., Gawronski, A., Pfeiffer, K., Kockler, H., Schilbach, L., & Vogeley, K. (2013). The investigation and differential diagnosis of Asperger Syndrome in adults. *Deutsches Ärzteblatt International, 110*(45), 755–763. https://doi.org/10.3238/arztebl.2013.0755

Lerman, D. C., Iwata, B. A., Shore, B. A., & Kahng, S. (1996). Responding maintained by intermittent reinforcement: Implications for the use of extinction with problem behavior in clinical settings. *Journal of*

Applied Behavior Analysis, 29(2), 153–171. https://doi.org/10.1901/jaba.1996.29-153

Lewis, L. F. (2017). "We will never be normal": The Experience of Discovering a Partner Has Autism Spectrum Disorder. *Journal of marital and family therapy.*

Lingsom, S. (2008). Invisible impairments: Dilemmas of concealment and disclosure *Scandinavian Journal of Disability Research, 10*(1), 2–16. https://doi.org/10.1080/15017410701391567

Livingston, L. A., Colvert, E., Bolton, P., & Happé, F. (2019). Good social skills despite poor theory of mind: exploring compensation in autism spectrum disorder. *Journal of Child Psychology and Psychiatry, 60*(1), 102–110. https://doi.org/10.1111/jcpp.12886

Mandy, W. (2019). Social camouflaging in autism: Is it time to lose the mask? *Autism, 23*(8), 1879–1881. https://doi.org/10.1177/1362361319878559

Marshack, K. J. (2009). *Life with a partner or spouse with Asperger Syndrome: Going over the edge? Practical steps to saving you and your relationship.* Autism Asperger Publishing Co.

Mashek, D. J., & Aron, A. (2004). *Handbook of closeness and intimacy.* Lawrence Erlbaum Associates. https://public.ebookcentral.proquest.com/choice/publicfullrecord.aspx?p=335513

McVey, A. J. (2019). The neurobiological presentation of anxiety in autism spectrum disorder: A systematic review. *Autism Research, 12*(3), 346–369. https://doi.org/10.1002/aur.2063

Mendes, E. (2015). *Marriage and lasting relationships with Asperger's Syndrome (Autism Spectrum Disorder): Successful strategies for couples or counselors.* Jessica Kingsley Publishers.

Millar-Powell, N., & Warburton, W. A. (2020). Caregiver burden and relationship satisfaction in ASD-NT relationships. *Journal of Relationships Research, 11.* https://doi.org/10.1017/jrr.2020.11

Milley, A., & Machalicek, W. (2012). Decreasing students' reliance on adults: A strategic guide for teachers of students with Autism Spectrum Disorders. *Intervention in School and Clinic, 48*(2), 67–75. https://doi.org/10.1177/1053451212449739

Milosavljevic, B., Carter Leno, V., Simonoff, E., Baird, G., Pickles, A., Jones, C. R. G., Erskine, C., Charman, T., & Happé, F. (2016). Alexithymia in adolescents with Autism Spectrum Disorder: Its relationship to internalising difficulties, sensory modulation and social cognition.

References

Journal of Autism and Developmental Disorders, 46(4), 1354–1367. https://doi.org/10.1007/s10803-015-2670-8

Moreno, S. J., Wheeler, M., & Parkinson, K. (2012). *The partner's guide to Asperger Syndrome.* Jessica Kingsley.

Murphy, L. (2015). Declarative Language. *RDIconnect* https://www.rdiconnect.com/declarative-language/

Patton, E. (2019). Autism, attributions and accommodations. *Personnel Review, 48*(4), 915–934. https://doi.org/10.1108/PR-04-2018-0116

Pearson, A., & Rose, K. (2021). A conceptual analysis of autistic masking: Understanding the narrative of stigma and the illusion of choice. *Autism in Adulthood, 3*(1), 1–9. http://doi.org/10.1089/aut.2020.0043

Portway, S. M., & Johnson, B. (2003). Asperger Syndrome and the children who 'don't quite fit'. *Early Child Development and Care, 173*(4), 435–443. https://doi.org/10.1080/0300443032000079113

Portway, S. M., & Johnson, B. (2005). Do you know I have Asperger's syndrome? Risks of a non-obvious disability. *Health, Risk & Society, 7*(1), 73–83. https://doi.org/10.1080/09500830500042086

Rearn, A. (2010). *Relationships and the importance of reciprocity.* http://www.goodtherapy.org/blog/relationship-reciprocity/

Reis, H. T., Lemay, E. P., & Finkenauer, C. (2017). Toward understanding understanding: The importance of feeling understood in relationships. *Social and Personality Psychology Compass, 11*(3). https://doi.org/10.1111/spc3.12308

Reiterer, S. M. (2018). *Exploring language aptitude : views from psychology, the language sciences, and cognitive neuroscience.* Springer. https://doi.org/10.1007/978-3-319-91917-1

Rench, C. (2014). *When Eros meets autos: Marriage to someone with autism spectrum disorder.* ProQuest Dissertations Publishing. http://search.proquest.com.ezproxy.ecu.edu.au/docview/1656449694?pq-origsite=summon&accountid=10675

Rodman, K. E. (2003). *Asperger's Syndome and adults ... Is anyone listening?.* Jessica Kingsley Publishers.

Sato, W., Kochiyama, T., Uono, S., Yoshimura, S., Kubota, Y., Sawada, R., Sakihama, M., & Toichi, M. (2017). Reduced gray matter volume in the social brain network in adults with Autism Spectrum Disorder. *Frontiers in human neuroscience, 11*, 395–395. https://doi.org/10.3389/fnhum.2017.00395

Simone, R. (2009). *22 things a woman must know if she loves a man with Asperger's Syndrome.* Jessica Kingsley Publishers.

Simons, H. F., & Thompson, J. R. (2009). Affective deprivation disorder: Does it constitute a relational disorder. *Affective deprivation disorder.*

Smith, R., Netto, J., Gribble, N. C., & Falkmer, M. (2020). 'At the end of the day, it's love': An exploration of relationships in neurodiverse couples. *Journal of Autism and Developmental Disorders.* https://doi.org/10.1007/s10803-020-04790-z

Stoddart, K. P. (2004). *Children, youth and adults with Asperger Syndrome: Integrating multiple perspectives.* Jessica Kingsley Publishers. https://ebookcentral.proquest.com/lib/ECU/detail.action?docID=290669

Tantam, D. (2012). *Autism Spectrum Disorders through the life span.* Jessica Kingsley Publishers.

Tsai, L. Y. (2013). Asperger's Disorder will be back. *Journal of Autism and Developmental Disorders, 43*(12), 2914–2942. https://doi.org/http://dx.doi.org/10.1007/s10803-013-1839-2

Vandervoort, D., & Rokach, A. (2003). Posttraumatic relationship syndrome: The conscious processing of the world of trauma. *Social Behavior and Personality, 31*(7), 675–685. http://findarticles.com/p/articles/mi_qa3852/is_200301/ai_n9213254/ (Provided by ProQuest Information and Learning Company)

Vandervoort, D., & Rokach, A. (2004). Abusive relationships: Is a new category for traumatization needed?. *Current Psychology, 23*(1), 68–76.

Vandervoort, D., & Rokach, A. (2006). Posttraumatic relationship syndrome: A case illustration. *Clinical Case Studies, 5*(3), 231–247. https://doi.org/10.1177/1534650104264934

Wang, Q. (2016). *Bridging the gap between declarative knowledge and procedural knowledge through metalinguistic corrective feedback.* [Doctoral dissertation, Boston University]. https://open.bu.edu/handle/2144/14568

Wilkinson, L. A. (2016, Thursday, June 30, 2016). Alexithymia, empathy, and autism. http://bestpracticeautism.blogspot.com.au/2012/02/alexithymia-empathy-and-autism.html

Zimmerman, M., Caroline, B., Iwona, C., & Kristy, D. (2018). Understanding the severity of depression: Which symptoms of depression are the best indicators of depression severity? *Comprehensive Psychiatry, 87,* 84–88.

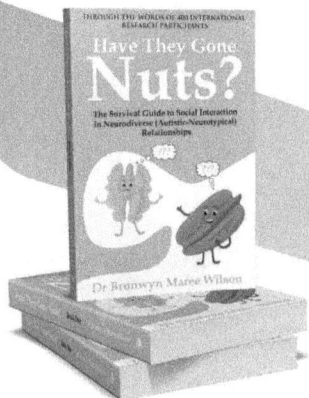

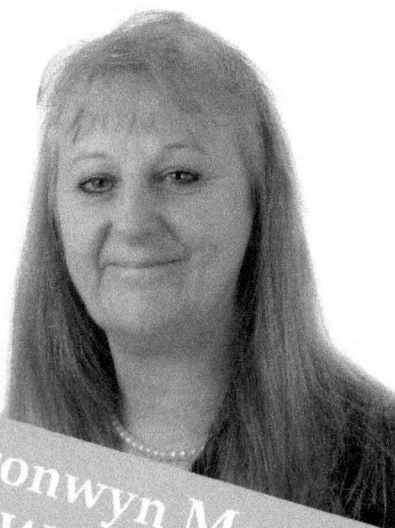

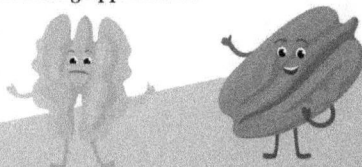

Free Bonuses

Growing The Knowing

Increase your knowing with bonus exclusive content

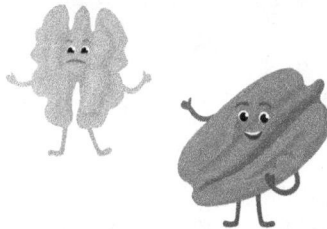

Life for people in neurodiverse relationships can be very different to those in conventional relationships. However, most of us did not know that a neurodiverse relationship was what we were getting into before we were in it. Many of us did not know until much, much later. Some of us have known for a few years. Some of us are just beginning to know. And some of us will never know. Even if we do know now, the neurodiverse relationship is still quite a mystery to most of us. Often, too confusing for words. No two are alike, just like no two typical relationships are alike. However, there are some common aspects. It is these common aspects that are important to know so that we can increase opportunities to grow in our relationship rather than grow out of it.

For access to bonus content that will assist you to grow your knowing, simply go to my website www.bronwilson. com, enter the password 'free articles' and follow the links to receive your extra bonus content directly to your inbox.

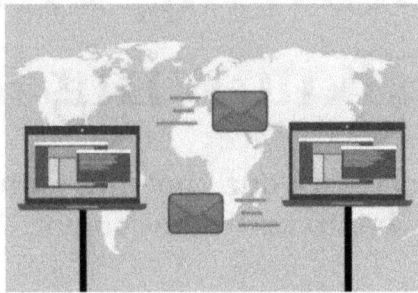

Increase your knowing with a ½ hour 'Ask the Expert' call

If reading this book has brought up questions or specific points and you would like expert guidance or more information, visit my website www.bronwilson.com, enter the password 'free strategy session' and follow the links to book a free one-on-one ½ hour Zoom session with me.

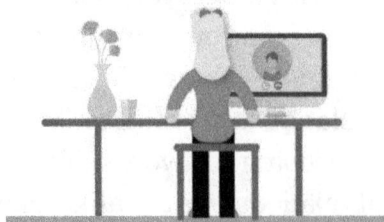

Growing The Knowing Learning Modules

12 Steps to Becoming a More Knowing You

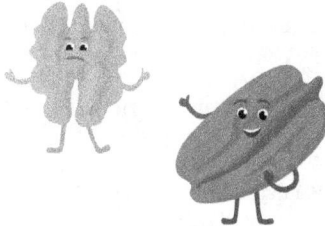

These learning modules are aligned to the book. Evidence suggests that ASC and NT adults have even greater differences compared to individuals from completely different cultures (Grigg, 2012; Rodman, 2003; Smith et al., 2020). When added together these differences collectively establish its own culture. The culture of the neurodiverse relationship, therefore, is like no other relationship. However, the more informed we are, the better prepared we are to make informed choices. For those who have a desire to know more, to dig deeper and to improve your understanding of the differences and difficulties specific to the neurodiverse relationship, these modules provide additional information on each topic covered in this book. Plus, a few extra bonus topics are also included. The more we know the more we grow. To get started go to the Growing the Knowing Learning Modules Tab on the website www.bronwilson.com

Have They Gone Nuts?

MODULE ONE: In the Beginning There Was Magic

- The Historical Context
- A Lost Generation
- Characteristics, Qualities and Fundamentals
- The Cognitive Differences
- Matters of Gender
- Matters of Attraction

MODULE TWO: The Mask Begins to Fall

- Masking: The Art of Camouflage
- Matters of Stigma
- Masking Increases Invisibility
- Constructing Normalcy, Perpetuating Invisibility
- Fear and Anxiety
- Intrinsic Motivation

MODULE THREE: The Language of Affection

- Social Learning
- Conveying Affection
- The Alexithymia Affect
- Expressing Feelings and Emotions
- Conversing About Personal Matters
- Deep and Meaningful Conversations

MODULE FOUR: A Collision of Needs

- Affection and Connection
- Company Without Connection
- Reciprocal Interaction
- Solitude Relieves Tensions
- Companionship
- Special Interests are a Refuge

MODULE FIVE: Facing A Different Page

- Needs Fulfilment
- Matters of Theory of Mind
- Matters of Executive Functions
- Matters Of Self and Other
- Mentalisation and Empathy
- A Predicament of Perceptions

MODULE SIX: Slaying the Dragon of Difference

- Dependence, Independence and Interdependence
- An Interpersonal Question and Response Shortfall
- Misinterpretations and Assumptions
- Prompting
- Guiding and Directing Conversations
- Conversation Preparation

MODULE SEVEN: A Permanent Millstone

- A Catch 22
- Conversation Avoidance
- The Perseveration Effect
- Achieving Responses
- Discussing Problems
- Dealing with Conflict

MODULE EIGHT: The Cycle Ensnares

- The Strength of Intermittent Schedules of Reinforcement
- Endlessly Prompting
- An Unrelenting Cycle
- Born from Conflict
- Cause of Conflict
- A Parental/Caretaker Role

MODULE NINE: The Cycle Multiplies

- Gottman's Four Horsemen
- Locked in Entangled Communication
- The Imitating Normalcy Cycle
- The Stonewalling Cycle
- The Help Seeking Cycle
- The Loss of Sense of Self Cycle

MODULE TEN: The Arrival of Cassandra

- Challenges of a Needs Deprivation
- The Cassandra Phenomenon
- The Impressions Others Hold
- Extended Family Systems
- Childish Allusions
- Notions of Irrationality

MODULE ELEVEN: Choices

- There is a Goldilocks Zone
- Thriving
- Depression and Looking Away
- Surviving
- Locking Out and Turning Away
- Deteriorating

MODULE TWELVE: Nuts and Bolts

- The Prompt Dependency Cycle
- The Implications of The Prompt Dependency Cycle
- The Outcomes of The Prompt Dependency Cycle
- The Keys That Unlock Healthier Options
- Two Models One Agenda
- A Preview of What is To Come

Acknowledgements

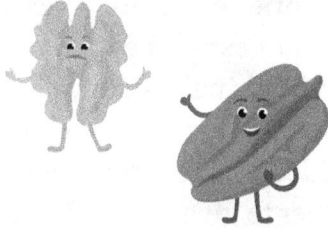

I express my sincere gratitude to each of my supervisors who supported me in my studies – Dr Wendi Beamish and Dr Steve Hay in the first, and Dr Susan Main, Dr John O'Rourke and Dr Deslea Konza in the second. Their professional and personal commitment, and their input and feedback, assisted in the realisation of research that I am honoured to have accomplished. Their valuable support has contributed to raising awareness of the unseen struggles of the population of people whose life challenges were explored in these studies.

A special mention goes to Professor Tony Attwood; a wise and knowledgeable supporter of my research journey, who, over quite a few years, has watched my personal and professional growth, while encouraging the development of my understanding of neurodiverse relationships.

I also thank God, who keeps me in His safe hands through all my dark hours (and there's been many), leading me through the circumstances and experiences that have allowed me to embark on this journey. After completing my first study, He kept me persisting through the second, to see them to their conclusions and then to authoring this book.

And lastly, but not at all least, I wish to thank all my participants who opened their lives to me with such forthrightness and honesty. They joined with me under a common cause, and willingly shared a part of themselves. Their collaboration, together with, the quality of data their candid input provided and contributions to the survey data, have worked together to give the studies and this associated book, depth and strength of meaning to make these projects the best that they could be.

My aspiration for this book is enhancement of knowledge regarding neurodiverse relationships in the wider community. The hope is that the understanding of those who provide the services, the programs, and the support, will be augmented, so they are better able to accomplish what they do best. The dream is to see an improvement in the lives, and a decline in the challenges faced, of those in neurodiverse relationships around the world.

Notes

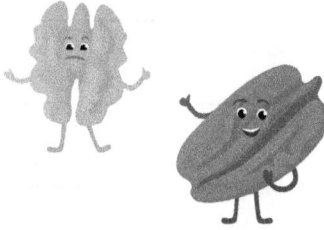

_____

_____

_____

_____

_____

_____

_____

_____

_____

Have They Gone Nuts?

Notes

_____

_____

_____

_____

_____

_____

_____

_____

_____

_____

_____

_____

_____

_____

_____

Have They Gone Nuts?

_____

_____

_____

_____

_____

_____

_____

_____

_____

_____

_____

_____

_____

_____

Notes

www.ingramcontent.com/pod-product-compliance
Lightning Source LLC
Chambersburg PA
CBHW032051020426
42335CB00011B/286